From Behaviour *To* Wellbeing

How Your Behaviour Can Help You Live A Good Life

Vinesh Sukumaran

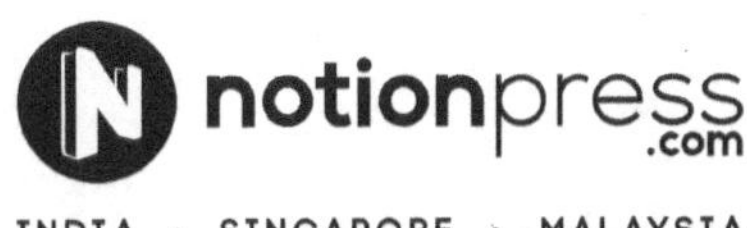

Notion Press

Old No. 38, New No. 6
McNichols Road, Chetpet
Chennai - 600 031

First Published by Notion Press 2018
Copyright © Vinesh Sukumaran 2018
All Rights Reserved.

ISBN 978-1-64324-478-5

Dedication

To my mother, my late father, my brother, sister-in-law and my two wonderful nieces.

CONTENTS

Contents

Contents

FOREWORD

Are you someone who is looking to achieve better health and happiness? Have you wanted to make positive changes in your life but have struggled to find the right tools to achieve your goals? Vinesh has done a great job of combining a variety of concepts into a simple and easy-to-use format with an emphasis on behavioural approaches to improving a person's quality of life and achieving the life you want.

Vinesh builds upon his experience as a personal and professional coach and writer. I met Vinesh as a graduate student taking some of my positive psychology courses at the University of Missouri. He has integrated concepts of positive psychology into his already strong set of skills as a coach and writer and has published articles in several popular magazines.

From his personal observations, he developed a useful approach by breaking down the concepts into simple and self-contained articles focused on a variety of concepts related to wellbeing. He places a strong emphasis on physical wellbeing and balances that with topics related to mindfulness, spirituality, happiness, emotional wellbeing and relationships.

By focusing on behavioural methods, he presents the information in a way that you can easily apply them in your life. He also utilises relatable examples from his own clients and adds in stories in parables to help illustrate key approaches. After reading this book, I was able to use the story he tells of the Zen master and the earthquake in my own practice as a clinical psychologist to help explain a concept to one of my patients.

He writes the material in specific and understandable ways, but the interventions have a great deal of support behind them. The information on gratitude stems from the field of positive psychology, where research supports the effectiveness of gratitude exercises in increasing happiness (Seligman, Steen, Park, & Peterson, 2005). His work on developing positive habits reminds me of the work by Charles Duhigg (2014) and the effective patterns he presents on how to make positive changes.

The section entitled "What Are You Constantly Telling Yourself" provides specific ways to identify and change your ways of thinking. His background is based on his training and experience in Neuro-Linguistic Programming (NLP), but also has many approaches grounded in Cognitive Behavioural Therapy (CBT). Some of the interventions are closely aligned to the tools to identify, challenge and change beliefs that I teach my clients using evidence-based treatments such as Cognitive Processing Therapy (CPT). It is very important for each of us to consider the specific thoughts and language that we speak to others or in our inner dialogue.

The challenge to be more positive is something illustrated in an old Native American story about a grandfather's lesson to his grandson. One day, a young boy goes to his grandfather and says, "I feel like I have two wolves fighting inside me." The grandfather replies, "You do indeed have two wolves fighting inside of you. One wolf is full of love, hope, humility, kindness and compassion. The other wolf is full of anger, envy, greed, self-pity, resentment, lies, and regret." The young boy thinks awhile and then asks, "But which one wins?" The wise grandfather says, "The one you choose to feed will win."

Like the story given above, many of the articles presented in this book are relatively short. This is done intentionally to allow you to study each one and take the time to implement the concepts into your life. As the author suggests, take the time to "lean into" each lesson, consider how to apply it to your own life, and use what works for you. If you are looking to improve your overall health, mental outlook, behaviours, spiritual life, and general wellbeing, I believe that you will find many useful approaches in this book.

Charles K. Hees, Ph.D.
Clinical Psychologist, Harry S. Truman
Memorial Veterans' Hospital.
Adjunct Instructor, University of Missouri.

References

Duhigg, C. (2014). *The power of habit: why we do what we do in life and business*. New York: Random House Trade Paperbacks, c2014.

Seligman, M. P., Steen, T. A., Park, N., & Peterson, C. (2005). Positive Psychology Progress: Empirical Validation of Interventions. American Psychologist, 60(5), 410-421.

PREFACE

A Good Way to Read This Book

This is not a book to be read in one shot or a book to be read from cover to cover. This is a book to lean into, reflect on what you've read and practice it before you lean in some more.

As a part of my work, I end up travelling a lot and therefore spend a lot of time in airports. Every time I see people at airports carrying books, I make it a point to notice how much of that book they've finished, either by looking at which part of the book they're reading or by looking at where the bookmark is placed. Over 90% of the time, most people are carrying a book that they've either just started or have read some but are still very close to the beginning. I think reading books is a dying habit and more and more people are moving into images, videos and perhaps reading just small snippets. I'd like this book to cater even to this generation in a way that suits them. So, it's divided into eight chapters, and each chapter has eight short articles. Chapters and articles are named to describe best what you'll find in them. The start of each chapter also has a snapshot that will give you a sense of the kind of articles covered under that chapter. So flip through the book, pick an article, the title of which interests you, and read it. Also, since there isn't a real narrative that runs through the book, you can pretty much pick random pieces from anywhere and read them.

In my work as an organisational development consultant, I've often met people who are trying to find their passion, shift careers, get better at something, be better managers or leaders, find happiness, find love, feel good about themselves and so on. People are in different stages of evolution on their journey to a good life. This book caters to a range of them. A friend once told me this joke. A boy gets back home from college and tells his mother, "Mom, I went on two dates today with two different women, and it feels so awesome." Just then the father walks into the house and tells his wife, "Honey, I got a hole in one today on the golf course, and it feels so awesome." As this couple and their son are sharing their excitement with each other, the grandfather comes out of the restroom and announces, "I had a good shit today, and it feels so awesome." What people are looking for and what makes them feel awesome varies based on where they are in their search for a good life. While for some, a good life might be about getting into great shape physically, for some others, it might be about feeling a sense of accomplishment about their work, and for some others, it might be about going beyond and finding spiritual meaning. Read what appeals to you and take back and use what strikes you the most.

ACKNOWLEDGEMENTS

There are a few people I want to thank, who chipped in generously at various stages in the writing of this book. First of all Dr. Charles Hees, who took the time out between his busy schedule at the hospital and university, to read through the entire book, give me valuable feedback as well as write a foreward that mattered. My dear friends Aadarsh Hariharan, Chaitanya Vembar and Rohit Nayak for reviewing the initial draft of the manuscript and giving me their comments and suggestions on anything from the phrasing of a single line and consistency of ideas to my voice as a writer. I owe it to Mr. Narasi Reddy, the Editor-in-chief of Stayfit Magazine, who encouraged me a few years ago to write an article every month and then publish them as a book, at some point. That really mattered, at a time when I'd just started writing for magazines in India. I'd also like to thank him for inducting me onto the panel of experts for Stayfit Magazine.

Almost twenty of the articles in this book are the outcome of long and animated discussions with my friend Silvia Riaño Rufilanchas over chilled beer and good food, about everything under the sun, from the Spanish bullfight and the works of Pedro Almodóvar to what makes the energy in Varanasi special. I want to thank her both for the good times and for the indelible mark that some of her ideas left on me. I want to thank three important people from the University of Missouri. Dr. Brandon Orr, my programme adviser, for building in me the competence of applying sport psychology and positive coaching. Dr. Graham Higgs for his insights on the nuances of positive psychology and his encouragement that made me want to write more. Sandra Sites from the college of education for answering all my questions, for her constant support and for just being there.

Finally, I want to thank all my clients, both individuals and organisations for what I've learnt through the sheer process of working with them and whose stories figure in every other page of this book.

INTRODUCTION

There are several interesting and sought-after ways to look at wellbeing out there. From what the Dalai Lama considers wellbeing, to what the University of Pennsylvania's Professor Martin Seligman says about it or what the Pope thinks wellbeing is. I've spent a big part of my adult life and pretty much my entire working life as a trainer, coach and consultant for organisations, helping people get better at what they do and start demonstrating the behaviours of their choice. It didn't matter what kind of an organisation I was training, which corporate executive I was coaching or which friend I was talking to at a café. One thing always remained. Every single person I've met was on a trip to experience more of the feelings and emotions that mattered the most to them at that point in time. It could be a student in her twenties wanting to feel loved, an experienced manager craving to feel successful, a middle-aged woman in a difficult marriage wanting to experience freedom again or even a stressed out but successful leader of a corporate giant wanting to experience real peace. If I was to sum this up in one word, I think 'Wellbeing' would be it. The one thing that everyone is after in some form or the other. Since this book is not meant just for the serious reader or student of psychology, I define wellbeing as a state of being happy, healthy and upbeat. Being fortunate and feeling good, if you like. In other words, living the good life. That's it. Every time I refer to wellbeing in this book, I'm talking about living the good life and that too based on your own standards.

Here's what professor Blaine Fowers from the University of Miami once said about the good life. In a 2011 piece, Blaine asked, "Do we really believe that the good life is a scientific question that, in the end, will produce a technical solution?"[1] The study of wellbeing would particularly benefit if it is furthered as a combined effort between scientists and researchers from various domains. As Compton and Hoffman put it, in their book on positive psychology, "A thorough understanding of happiness requires input from psychologists, sociologists, philosophers, artists, cultural anthropologists, theologians, and many others. A complete understanding of wellbeing needs science and wisdom; group statistics and individual lives; objectivity and empathy; understanding and compassion."[2] I've focused to a large extent on physical wellness since a lot of us see that as the hallmark of wellbeing. Understanding human behaviour and the role it plays in moving you towards where you want to be might just be your ticket to greater wellbeing. By the way, I've never felt that people need to make changes to their lives or that they need to hit certain success, prosperity or happiness targets. I think people are perfect just the way they are. This book is about realising exactly why even some people who want to get happier and live the good life end up not being able to do it.

I cover here, a lot of the nuances of human behaviour. There are two things that mostly interest anyone who's studying behaviour. First, the unique dimensions of behaviour. It always fascinates people when they see a behaviour that is so unimaginable that they go "I don't get it," "Why would someone do that?," "How does someone do that?," "That's crazy!," "Really? She did that?." Such behaviours are pondered over, talked about, even discussed to death, and every psychologist worth his salt loves to give his or her own explanation for the behaviour. The second thing that interests people are patterns of behaviour. There is something about the predictability of a behaviour that makes people grin and say to themselves "I knew it," "I just knew it," "Oh yes! I knew that was coming," "I'm not surprised," "what else did you expect?." And, obviously, in between these two extremes, of exclusive behaviours and obvious behaviours, there must be something else. That, I think, is what this book is mostly full of. The kind of behaviours that you instinctively knew all along, but never bothered naming or defining. Just knowing this puts you in a much better place as far as directing yourself towards your own version of the good life is concerned.

IS THERE SOMETHING BEYOND WELLBEING?

A SNAPSHOT

This chapter questions if wellbeing is really a pursuit for you at all. If it isn't, then what is? There are a lot of answers to that question which inevitably lead to some dimension of wellbeing. From good looks to a good space to live in to spiritual progress. And there are some who don't believe in pursuing anything in particular because they believe that it's all fate or destiny. I've discussed some of these here and looked at the clear advantages and shortcomings of certain things that we are after in life. I've noticed that it's quite challenging to change somebody's mind if it's firmly set on something. A senior corporate executive who's decided that he wants to become a CEO and then make more money and then buy more things and only then be happy, is like a Toro Bravo in a Spanish bullring face to face with an unarmed matador. He might get a heart attack trying, but will not settle for going directly to happiness, even though he has a choice to. This chapter brings together my reading and insights on the purpose and meaning in life along with the hollowness that I've seen in some of the most successful people I've met. People who've achieved what most would consider a raging success but they still felt incomplete inside. This chapter also draws from my interest in art and how it can be used as a vestibule to a good life.

WHAT EMOTIONS ARE YOU CHASING?

Irrespective of which industry, which profession, which stage of your career or life you're in, or even if you aren't part of any industry, profession or career, one thing remains common to everything you do. A positive intention. In essence, everything that anybody does has a positive intention. This is not to be mistaken for the fact that everything that anybody does is done for the greater good of humanity or the world. That's obviously not true. The point is that when anyone does anything, they do it with the positive intention of getting a particular outcome. What often gets muddled is that people may not have absolute clarity about what exactly they want to achieve and what things might look like after they achieve it. It's safe to say that often in life, we end up aiming for and achieving things, which we later realise, are not what we actually wanted.

This reminds me of the wonderful old story by Lewis Carroll, *Alice in Wonderland*. There's a point in the story where Alice is walking in Wonderland and is looking for direction. On the bough of a tree, she sees this beautiful cat called the Cheshire cat. A conversation between the cat and Alice goes something like this:

Alice: Would you tell me, please, which way I ought to go from here?

Cheshire Cat: That depends a good deal on where you want to get to.

Alice: I don't much care where.

Cheshire Cat: Then it doesn't matter which way you go

Alice: … So long as I get somewhere.

Cheshire Cat: Oh, you're sure to do that, if you only walk long enough.

Though this was supposed to be a book for children, there are amazing lessons for people from all walks of life in it. For example, the above conversation makes it crystal clear that even in life, if you don't know where you want to get to, then pretty much any road will take you there.

One of the best things that you can do for yourself is to ask yourself this most relevant question:

What do you want in life?

Or better still. What do you actually want in life?

I've asked these questions to many people during coaching sessions, and some responses I've heard are:

❖ A better job
❖ A higher salary
❖ Marriage
❖ A baby
❖ A big house
❖ A BMW
❖ An ideal life partner
❖ A fat bank balance, etc.

These are obviously genuine answers. Yet, they might not be the things that people actually want in life. Unfortunately, there are many who might spend an entire lifetime pursuing them, not even getting past their allure. If you scratch the surface a little more, you'll realise that the reason someone wants a fat bank balance, a big house or an ideal life partner is to achieve something larger in life and some of them have given me these answers straight away. Things like,

- ❖ A feeling of security
- ❖ The sense of pride
- ❖ Pure joy
- ❖ Excitement
- ❖ Happiness
- ❖ Peace of mind
- ❖ Love, etc.

These feelings or emotions are what most people are actually after and that is what underlies most of our goals. They're essentially what all human beings are trying to experience in life.

Just realising this helps you shift gears from chasing momentary excitement to experiencing sustained positive emotions. This shift typically gives your positive intentions a new edge and therefore makes you take actions that could save you months, years and sometimes an entire lifetime of toil and effort.

THE MYTH ABOUT GOOD-LOOKING PEOPLE

I recently had a somewhat animated discussion with an image consultant about the impact of good looks on corporate and social success. Her point of view was simple and direct. She said that good-looking people find it easier to get a job, keep a job and grow in that job to senior positions. She also added that another natural outcome of being good looking is that you end up having a better circle of friends and, in turn, a better social life. Obviously, she isn't alone in the "good-looking people have better lives" bandwagon.

Various universities have conducted research on the benefits of good looks. A Yale University study[3] found that attractive men and women earn more than their average-looking counterparts. Another Harvard University study[4] found that investors were more likely to put money into businesses if the man making the pitch is handsome. There is also a study that was conducted at the University of Zurich[5] that correlates higher levels of human endurance with good looks.

This bias towards good looks is not just confined to the corporate world. Its reach spreads way beyond that into various social settings. Someone once told me that in many parts of the world it's almost impossible to find an extremely beautiful woman doing the job of sweeping streets or clearing trash. It might be equally challenging in many parts of the world to find an extremely handsome gentleman doing a low end, menial job. It's almost as if merely being good looking assures you a better job and a better position in society. For the most part, you might also observe in social circles that it's the good-looking people who are more likely to be the social butterflies. As I mentioned earlier, this is the point of view that the image consultant had, and it is one that gets established by the popular media's huge focus on good looks. Whether it's the age-old print medium, banners, billboards, television or the internet, as long as there are visuals, there is bound to be a focus on good-looking people. The popular media are almost addicted to good looks. How often do you see an ugly-looking man or woman in a fashion, cosmetic or clothing ad? It's almost as difficult to find models who are not good looking even in ads for products like cars, chocolates, soft drinks, mobile phones or home accessories. People playing the lead roles in commercial movies are almost always good looking. On the face of it, this entire obsession with good looks could seem overwhelming, and in a world of bariatric surgeries, Botox and anti-ageing, people like the image consultant I was speaking to are actually not out of place.

While the media might flood us with visuals and slogans to keep the importance of good looks in our active consciousness, if we took a step back, we'd realise that there's also the other side. There is an inner side to humanity that overshadows the outer synthetic covering and gloss. With some amount of reflection and recollection, anyone will see that in almost every field, there are numerous examples of people who don't necessarily look good physically but who are extremely attractive because of who they are. Even Hollywood and the silver screen, in general, has numerous stars who are admired by their endless number of fans for qualities beyond looks, like their dialogues, their acting skills and sometimes even the characters they played.

There is a point in everyone's life when the importance of qualities like inner peace, satisfaction and happiness outweighs the importance of good looks and physical attraction. People around the world are beginning to realise that merely having good looks is not everything. In fact, lead researcher James McNulty of the University of Tennessee[6] talks about how absolute beauty is important only in the early stages of a relationship for young couples and that the role of physical attractiveness in well-established partnerships, such as marriage, is somewhat of a mystery. Also, anyone who's interviewed some of the billionaires or successful people in any field, seeking to know their secrets to a good life, will tell you that good looks rarely figures on any of the lists.

While physical attractiveness and good looks are important, they are only a part of the whole and are in no way conclusive indicators of a better life in any respect. When you first see a person from a distance, the only data points you have are likely to be the ones pertaining to their physical appearance. The way they are dressed, their skin tone, physique or in which direction they're looking. As you keep observing the person, you start to detect more data points related to the way the person walks, moves, gestures or even their overall behaviour. If you begin to actually interact with the person, you're likely to be swamped with data points related to the person's profession, background, interests, attitude, values or even beliefs. If you like some of these elements that you discover from your interaction and if they resonate with your own, the person might start looking better to you. I mean this literally. Here are a few examples. An average-looking person might start looking great to you after you discover that he or she is a self-made business tycoon or is the author of a few bestsellers. On the contrary, even a good-looking person might start looking average when you realise that he or she reeks or doesn't have a sense of humour. You are likely to find an average-looking person better looking if you get to know that that person has similar ideologies and values as you do. Several mediocre-looking individuals start to look better in the eyes of the world after attaining high levels of success in their fields or after striking glory of any kind.

As a matter of fact, there are several examples in the world of people (celebrities included) who might not even appear on the actual radar screen of good looks but who are rated as good looking in public opinion polls mostly because of their achievements and other qualities. Certainly, this is a rating that they would not have received in the absence of their other achievements or qualities. High levels of competence and expertise have a kind of magnetism that goes beyond physical features and appearance. Intelligence, a sense of humour and genius are attractive at levels that are far beyond the clothes you wear or your complexion. Kindness, compassion and niceness build relationships that far outlive momentary bonds of infatuation or one-night stands. Good looks can't possibly be the secret to fame, fortune and glory. The real perks of this generation go to individuals who capitalise on their biggest strengths, whatever they are. Barring a few fields in the sphere of entertainment like modelling, in most others, good looks might be nothing more than just an add-on. With the direction in which the world is headed, there is an increasing number of jobs and entire fields with limited direct human interaction. This phenomenon is only going to increase in the future with a majority of our communication shifting to emails, mobile phones and texting.

These were my closing comments to the image consultant while she still stuck on to her own perspective. I'm sure we might have found each other far more attractive had we agreed on each other's points of view.

THE LINK BETWEEN MONEY AND SPIRITUALITY

If you had to choose between two options, becoming more spiritual or having more money, what would you choose? Where would you put your money? On spirituality or on wealth? Or shall we say, where does your heart lie? In spirituality or in money? What's more important than making a choice between the two is to understand how one and in turn the other could impact your life. Will having more money make you more spiritual or will it take away from your level of spirituality?

In the year 1943, Abraham Maslow in his paper 'A Theory of Human Motivation' proposed a theory in psychology called the Maslow's Hierarchy of Needs[7]. In this theory, he represented human needs at different levels in a pyramid with the most basic physiological needs right at the bottom and moving upwards to other needs like the need for safety, love or belonging, esteem and finally the need for self-actualisation right at the top of the pyramid.

A need to make spiritual progress or attain self-realisation is linked more to the self-actualisation need which surfaces strongly only after the other lower needs are met. How having money aligns with this theory is that it helps you meet all your basic needs and perhaps even helps you attain the need for esteem or self-respect. Having satisfied all these needs, the next logical level is to try and fulfil the self-actualisation need, and one of the prominent dimensions of this need is making spiritual progress. Some people (not all) who don't have adequate money might end up spending a lifetime trying to fulfil their need for self-esteem or the need to feel a sense of belongingness or sometimes even just trying to ensure safety and security in life. This short-sightedness might end up curtailing the spiritual progress that they could have made had their basic needs been met.

Now I don't want to sound as if money is the passport to spiritual growth. It isn't. But what's worth noting is that having more money almost eternally has been linked with having more material possessions. Many of the super-rich realise at some point that merely making more money and accumulating more material assets has real limitations. "What next?" is the big question. Especially when you can buy or own almost anything that you can think of, areas like spirituality particularly start to seem more meaningful. Some of the richest people in the world also end up being the biggest philanthropists for precisely this reason. While quite a few of the rich and affluent shift their interests to spirituality due to the sheer boredom of material pursuits, many of them actually see spirituality as an area that will help them live a more fulfilling and satisfied life. The song *Can't Buy Me Love* by the 1960's band The Beatles has a useful message for all of us. There's a line in the song that goes "… I don't care too much for money, and money can't buy me love." Unfortunately, there are many of us in this world who realise this a shade too late in life.

It's not uncommon to find people in the urban working world who spend most of their lives slogging and making money or amassing wealth till one day they are affected by an incurable disease or have lost a loved one. They realise at this point that no amount of money or material possessions can cure them or bring their loved ones back to life. There are a lot of things like love, happiness, peace of mind, contentment, etc., that money can't buy. Another very common phenomenon among all sections of society is that as people start to get older, they realise that the money and wealth that they were working so hard to put together won't help them eliminate loneliness or cure insomnia. Nor are money and wealth things that they are going to take with them when they kick the bucket. This realisation often pushes people to explore spirituality. There's no point lying on your death bed thinking of how you needn't have worked so hard after all and could have spent more time with your family instead of at airport lounges.

It's not always that people wait to start growing old to realise the importance of spirituality. There are several cases where this realisation hits individuals earlier on in life. T. Harv Eker[8], the author of *Secrets of the Millionaire Mind*, talks about something interesting in his seminars. He says that the best thing about becoming a millionaire or getting rich is not the money itself; it's who you have to become to make that money. In other words, to increase your wealth creation potential, you have to become a bigger, better person in many ways. A strong part of this personal growth is the spiritual dimension, be it a meditation practice, belief in God or even appreciation for the good things in life or gratitude. Many of the rich and famous realise that a strong spiritual dimension in their lives will actually help them achieve greater fame and fortune. In the 1992 American Music Awards, when Will Smith and Jazzy Jeff won the award for the best rap album, they came up on stage to receive the award, and Will Smith highlighted the importance of being grounded in spite of any kind of success or celebrity status. Many a times, even money comes with a price tag. The success, fame, glory, hectic lifestyle or stress related to stardom are part and parcel of your earning potential. To deal with these effectively, many turn to spirituality.

Lastly, spirituality is a great leveller. Your bank balance or net worth might have an impact on steering you towards spirituality but might have little to do with the quality of the spiritual journey thereafter. In that sense, spirituality could be an absolute leveller. The quality of your spiritual experience has nothing to do with how much money you have. Whether it is the blissful experience of a soft breeze hitting your face by a meadow in the countryside or a life-transforming realisation that you have while in a deep meditative trance. As a matter of fact, for many who belong to the not so financially sound segments of society, a spiritual practice or experience is something that takes them beyond money, status and power. Likewise, for the wealthy segments of society, spirituality and the related higher experiences are things that are beyond what their money can possibly give them.

THE "MINE IS BIGGER THAN YOURS" PHENOMENON IN SPIRITUALITY

Just the word 'spirituality' conjures up all kinds of references, implications and ideas in people's minds. From the spiritual character of thought to the incorporeal, from delicately refined to sacred or devotional and from the essence of religion to the supernatural. Irrespective of what spirituality means to a person, there is a sense among those driven by spirituality to get to a more spiritual level and make progress towards a spot of attainment. If this was not true, the person might simply not be driven by the spiritual pursuit and would be pursuing something else instead. This is the basis of what I call the "mine is bigger than yours" phenomenon in spirituality. Like other concepts like the "peacock tail effect"[9] in evolutionary psychology, the word 'bigger' here doesn't merely refer to size. It refers to a higher level of sophistication, eliteness, some form or the other of superiority and a greater degree of authenticity or quality if you like. Apart from the base ideas of superiority of one religion over another, this phenomenon shows itself up in multiple ways especially in an age of power wellness and power spirituality. Here are some ways in which you might see the "mine is bigger than yours" phenomenon manifest itself in the world of spirituality.

The Inner Circle Syndrome

Spiritual leaders all over the world might have experienced this at some point of time. In many ashrams or retreats, there are likely to be one or two key spiritual leaders who are at the so-called helm of affairs. It's quite common in such situations, to see some followers losing focus on their spiritual path and aiming to get closer to the Guru or the main spiritual leader, to become part of their inner circle. There are some who even go to the extent of wanting to be the "favourite" follower or disciple. While there is nothing particularly wrong with this, it simply isn't what a spiritual journey is all about.

The Journey Destination Conflict

There are several roads that lead to the destination of the spiritual experience and many a times, the spiritual experience is the road itself. There's an unsaid clash of different mindsets here. While one set of people pursue spirituality to get to a final point of bliss, enlightenment or whatever you choose to call it, there is another set that attributes more importance to the spiritual journey rather than the destination. Of course, there is a third group that gives equal importance to the spiritual journey and the destination or sees no difference between the two. While each of these mindsets has some kernel of truth in it, it certainly doesn't establish the superiority of one mindset over the other. All it establishes is that people need to pursue spirituality based on what works for them.

The Duration Myth

The duration factor plays a crucial role in people's perceptions of a spiritual practice. While there's no debate on the fact that with time and practice one gets better at anything including with a spiritual practice, the duration is not certainly an indicator of spiritual progress. It's almost as if a quick path or easy access to a spiritual experience is not real or authentic. There are some who have had profound spiritual experiences in their very first attempt or class while there are some who have had a life-changing spiritual experience on a particular day after many years of practice, and there are still others who might have been on a trek in the mountains or just watching children play at a park and had an awesome spiritual awakening. Another dimension of the duration myth is related to the actual duration of the spiritual practice itself. For instance, many meditators see the ability to meditate for extended periods at a stretch to be more advanced than meditating for a few minutes a day. Though it might require a certain amount of practice and ability to even sit in the same position for more than an hour, it's certainly not an indicator of the quality or level of one's spirituality.

The Experience Trap

It's likely in any spiritual practice for people to have interesting experiences at different points. These experiences could be anything from a feeling of immense peace, to stillness or even feeling the presence of God in one's own sweet way. What mostly gets missed out is that spirituality is beyond these experiences. Unfortunately, many individuals get sucked into or sometimes even get addicted to these experiences. Worse still, people even equate the nature of the experience to spiritual progress. This is nothing more than a ludicrous way of reducing spirituality to a mere set of experiences.

A Spiritual Experience Needs to Be Complex

No, it does not. There are talks by some spiritual gurus that specifically state that if someone can describe a spiritual experience to you, then it is not a real spiritual experience because a true spiritual experience cannot be described in words. While an extended spiritual experience could be more difficult to explain than some simpler feelings and emotions, it's certainly not a metric of the calibre of the experience itself. It is perfectly possible for someone with a good enough vocabulary to explain the range of feelings and emotions that he experienced during a spiritual trip, and that does not take away from the quality or genuineness of that experience. On the other hand, it is also true that some deep spiritual experiences are nothing more than simple feelings like gratitude, humility, peace, love and togetherness which are well understood by most people.

Worshipping The Unknown

This is an extension of the previous point and a cornerstone of sorts when it comes to the entire idea of spiritual comparison. In many parts of the world, the whole idea of spirituality leans heavily on God, mythology and other beliefs. A belief is something that one has conviction in and decides to take for granted; something that is held as true despite the odds. So the concept of belief is foundational to spirituality. Even with respect to spiritual experiences, our treatment is no different. When someone has a spiritual experience that is inexplicable, unclear and perhaps incomprehensible, it is given greater importance than an experience that is more direct and clearly understood. For instance, when a person is involved in a spiritual practice and experiences a series of colours in front of them when sitting with closed eyes, feels a burst of energy from their gut and transcends into a space of peace and tranquillity like never before, it is treated as a blessed event. Perhaps, one that is showered on the person by the almighty and one that the person was "lucky" to have experienced. On the contrary, if someone sits down for a spiritual practice but gets lost in thought for the next hour thinking of his or her school days and school friends and feels great and light in the head at the end of it, it is treated as a daydream. This is also the same reason why an out-of-body experience is treated as a more spiritual experience than the feeling of bliss while lying on your couch on a Sunday afternoon reading your favourite book.

No spiritual experience is better or worse. Running is no superior to jogging or walking and vice versa. They're all different experiences and have their own place in the scheme of things. The same applies to spirituality. To grow spiritually, all you need to do is stay on your spiritual path and experience. Just be at it. Stepping out of that and focusing on ideas like the superiority of the spiritual experience and spiritual tenure will take you several steps back or at best, keep you marking time.

ARE FATE AND WELLBEING RELATED?

If you are expecting to read here about whether you are destined to be in a state of good health and wellbeing, then read no more. The only point that I want to really highlight here is how a belief in fate or the lack of it could impact your wellbeing and perhaps all areas of your life.

Incidents like the 9/11 attacks in the U.S., the tsunami, and earthquakes in Haiti and Nepal are great tragedies of our times and one sometimes wonders about the implications of such a large number of people getting wiped out in one shot. Among them were people who worked out, who didn't work out, people who smoked, who didn't smoke, people who were hardcore meat eaters, vegetarian or vegan. This raises some fundamental questions in people's minds:

- ❖ What is the point of trying to live healthy?
- ❖ Is there any sense in waking up early, working out or practising a fitness regime?
- ❖ Is there a larger force controlling all of us puppets?

While it's only natural and healthy to have these thoughts, the problem is when you let them tie you down or cause you to hand over the controls of your life to something like fate that you're not sure of. The real danger is if you start living an unhealthy lifestyle, develop addictions and stop nourishing your mind and an earthquake or tsunami doesn't hit.

If fate is removed out of this picture, then the only thing left to do is to take responsibility, where You hold the controls and accept the fact that the only reason for your poor health or mediocre level of fitness or supreme wellbeing is You. There is simply no question about the difficulty of people born with disabilities or into bad circumstances or even into the wrong part of the planet. But by refusing to take control, you're refusing to grow up and grow out of your circumstances. Despite your disabilities and circumstances, you can tap into a state of incredible wellbeing. Especially since we all know that wellbeing is beyond just working out in the gym or going for a run. The quadriplegic Nick Vujicic[10] is a classic example of this and his movie *No Arms, No Legs, No Worries* embodies it.

Another popular phenomenon in the same ballpark is for people to take credit for their achievements and blame their shortcomings on fate or something out of their control. If you have a six-pack, then you worked for it; if you have a beer belly, then it's the genetics. The lottery industry is filled with people who rely on luck, chance and fate instead of working towards realising their dreams. That's exactly why, for every lottery winner, there are a million losers.

There will always be things that are out of your control as the past has shown and the future is likely to show. You better not sit back and say "It's fate" because that hardly helps. Moving ahead and doing something about it does.

A belief in fate is best used for things that you actually can't control, so that you make your peace with it a lot more easily, be it wellbeing or anything else. Fate is not a dartboard to throw arrows at as a result of your own incompetence.

ZEN AND THE ART OF DECLUTTERING

A friend of mine who lived in my city for several years recently shifted back to her country, and I was on the cusp of the shifting process. It was shocking to see how much stuff someone can have with them that they might never use and sometimes have never used at all. One of the interpretations of the Pareto principle[11] says that 80% of the time, we might keep wearing just 20% of the clothes in our wardrobes. I think this pretty much applies to all other things that we stock up for eternal non-usage. In my view, decluttering is not just about getting rid of junk but also about getting rid of your baggage. Here's how you could go about doing it in a progressive fashion.

Start by looking into your shelves, wardrobes, attics, draws, lofts and closets. Take out everything that you haven't used in a year and are not likely to use in the next year and put it into a large bag that will form part of the junk that is "to be disposed of." Keep doing this till you can't find anything that falls under the 'to be disposed of' category. Then get rid of that bag by selling the stuff in it, donating it to an orphanage or giving it to someone who you think might need it. This is not a suggestion to get rid of something really precious like your ancestral family jewellery or something like your wedding gown that has real sentimental value even if you might never wear it ever again. If you're one of those people who treats every pin and empty perfume bottle like it was your wedding gown, then try this. Take out those things that you're trying to hold on to anyway and put them into a 'to be disposed of' bag. Zip up this bag and keep it aside for six months. In six months, if you never use any of the things in that bag, then without a second thought, pick up that bag and get rid of it. If you did use any of the things in the bag in six months, then keep just those things aside for later disposal. While getting rid of useless things is just the first step, it's a great way of not just clearing up physical space in your house but also mental space in your head. It's like the difference between sitting at an overcluttered and dusty desk versus sitting at an organised and clean desk. Decluttering helps you think more clearly.

The second step of decluttering is to look at how you spend your time throughout the day. Stop doing all those things that you do that have no meaning or purpose and don't add any value to your life. Whether it's talking on the phone unnecessarily, mindless watching of television or channel-surfing, cyber-loafing and just jumping from one website to another, or checking out what everyone under the sun is up to on Facebook. Just stopping these activities will free out time to do the things that really matter to you, that make you feel good and that actually add value to your life.

Thirdly, start decluttering people. We all have people in our lives who matter to us and who care and reciprocate our feelings and gestures toward them. They are the ones you should be spending most of your time with. Scan your life and identify those people who you might be talking to or interacting with on a regular basis, but who are an absolute waste of your time. There could be people who just talk to unload their burdens on you, some who call you only when they need something and are never there for you when you need them and some others who want someone to while away their time with and in the process sap your energy dry. The idea is not to call these people up and sever all relationships with them in one shot. Rather than pulling the plug abruptly, slowly stop entertaining them and keep your interaction with them to the minimum. This will either keep them at that minimum interaction level or cause them to fade away on their own.

If you've managed to do this much, then you've really made headway, and I'm sure the quality of your life has increased several fold. Just to add some whipped cream and cherry to your decluttering exercise, you could also try mental decluttering. Watch your thoughts throughout the day and start identifying all the useless, unproductive and unconstructive thoughts that you have. If you like, you could start journaling your habitual thoughts throughout the day. After a couple of days, if you look back at what you've captured, you'll clearly be able to identify the useless and unsupportive thoughts that you're indulging in. This self-awareness really helps because then, every time you catch yourself thinking one of those lousy thoughts, you could quickly and deliberately replace it with a positive one. I've tried each of these tips myself and have also helped my clients use them. In the beginning, it's easier said than done. But with practice, you'll start to find it a lot easier to do, and the benefits of decluttering your mind and dwelling on the positive and supportive thoughts far outweigh the benefits of merely clearing out the clutter from your closet.

USE ART TO CLEAR YOUR MIND

I once asked a distinguished art therapist in Japan, "What is it about art that gives it its therapeutic quality?" She said, "It sometimes silences your mind and if required empties it and brings it back to its truest and most natural state of being." She, of course, went on to tell me, how she had used art to relieve people of milder challenges like stress, body aches and worries as well as cure people of more serious diseases like cancer, heart ailments, depression, stroke and bipolar disorder.

In a world of rat races and reducing human interaction shrouded by pokes, likes, Whatsapp messages and tweets, the run-of-the-mill human mind is in anything but its natural state. Expression is a very basic human instinct. But due to the nature of corporate hierarchies, social conditioning and sometimes even governments, people are forced to curb these instincts. There's a lot of mental clutter that accumulates as a result of things that we do throughout the day. For example, people who get back home after a hectic day and fall asleep after a heavy dinner, accumulate all the pent-up stress in their systems. People who have unresolved arguments, fights and difficult relationships of all kinds, carry feelings of guilt, anger and revenge for months and sometimes years. Feelings and emotions like regret, failure, sadness and discontent get bottled up into mental clutter that later translate quite effectively into disease and pestilence.

So let me plunge in and get to the essence of what it is about art that will help in clearing your mind. Even for those who aren't directly involved in the creation of art, merely going into a good art gallery to see an art exhibition or display of paintings will help. The silence of the art gallery, the beauty of the pieces displayed and the stillness and serene energy around helps in slowing the mind down from its daily breakneck pace.

For those involved in the creation of a piece of art or are willing to embark on that journey, here are just a few ways in which you might benefit.

Being Here and Now

One of the phenomenal qualities of creating a piece of art is that it forces you to step into the present. Since most of our mental fog is either about the future or the past, merely being in the present for an extended period of time helps in creating the mental space required to process other information later. While there are several other activities that could offer the same benefit, art does so in a cajoling and non-threatening way, especially if approached in the right manner. Don't start doing a painting with a specific finishing time in mind or a very accurate visual outcome. Go with the flow. Even if you have no clue about what you're going to paint, allow the blankness of the page or canvass to guide you. Let your intuition and instincts guide your hand

and keep following it. If you're not a person who is used to starting without a definite image or goal in mind, try one of the following:

- ❖ Try to get that image completely wrong in all possible ways and enjoy the process of doing it.
- ❖ Try to create that entire image with scribbles and splashes of colour rather than with well-defined lines. This will really help you loosen up.
- ❖ Try the minimalist approach. Reduce the image to its bare essence by stripping it off anything unnecessary. Ask yourself what would be the simplest form of the image and just paint that.

People have learnt valuable lessons about going with the flow, not being perfectionists and simplifying their own lives by following some of the above techniques. Moreover, staying invested in the creation of a painting for an hour is equivalent to an hour of mindfulness meditation.

Emotional Decluttering

Art, especially with the use of colour, has direct access to the emotional part of your brain. The amygdala, an almond-shaped mass of nuclei located deep within the temporal lobe of the brain is responsible for several of our emotions and motivations, especially the more rudimentary ones. It is the seat of several of the intense emotions like fear, anger and pleasure. Also, the right side is the more intuitive, imaginative and creative side of the brain. Art greatly stimulates the amygdala and involves the use of the right brain in general. With the use of different colours, with the creation of vivid images and with the exercising of intuition, a lot of the bottled up emotional pressure is released. This will give you a renewed sense of being able to deal with your life's situation and challenges. Mild headaches to severe migraines have been cured as a result of emotional decluttering.

Feeling Good

As a result of trying to meet strict deadlines, following set and rigid processes and doing routine work, many have lost the sense of how it feels to create something new. Painting or sketching will put you back in touch with your ability to create. It clears the mind off the monotony of repetition and ushers in new energy like a whiff of fresh air. The feeling of having created something beautiful and impressive brings in a sense of accomplishment that you can carry to other areas of your life. Many who pursue art even develop a serious interest in it and become part of a new circuit of friends and associates. This in itself could be a stimulating experience both with respect to how much you end up learning from each other as well as being exposed to a host of new ideas and ways of looking at life.

Back to Basics

As mentioned earlier, one of the basic instincts of the human mind that is curbed in the world today is the instinct of expression. Art creates a clear outlet for expression. Drawing, painting, etching, scribbling, splashing colours, etc., are all modes of expression. Art will help you express yourself in a manner that is more fundamental and intrinsic. It's normal for people who are involved in any form of art to feel light and rejuvenated after taking a piece to completion. Many who have been involved in some form of art long enough even develop a deep appreciation for doing art for art's sake. A painting is created purely to express themselves in a manner that is most real and natural. The process of expression is embraced to its fullest for the sake of the experience rather than for social approval or to impress the world around them. People who've understood this also carry this mindset wherever they go. They become more interested in experiencing life rather than missing the actual experience and clicking pictures of it to share and broadcast.

While most of what is discussed here is in reference to the fine art of painting or sketching, the same applies to any other form of art. Music, dance, any of the martial arts, writing and photography are all popular examples. In short, it applies to methods and techniques of art collectively and to any product of human creativity.

EVERYTHING IN LIFE HAS AN EXPIRY DATE

I recently met a friend after several years, and when we sat down at this restaurant for dinner, like all old friendships, it was great to catch up and revisit old times and realise how much we had in common and knew about each other. What was also clear was that despite all our commonalities, we had also grown quite differently as individuals and in that sense, though nothing much had changed, in reality, a lot had changed. Like this friend of mine had stopped drinking, stopped smoking, stopped eating meat and had turned completely vegan. He told me all this in a really matter of fact way. That was really where this article began. It made me realise that everything has its time and validity period.

We grow into and out of things as we grow older. There was a time in my life when, if I didn't go out for a big party on the 31st of December, the New Year's celebration just didn't feel complete. That idea expired long ago, and I don't go out and party likes a rockstar anymore. But looking back, I'm glad I went to those parties and celebrations at a time when they made that much sense to me. Another common predicament I keep hearing about is how people have to make sudden changes in their lifestyles. A sudden diagnosis of a heart disease or cancer or sometimes even diabetes or hypertension immediately slaps a strict diet and lifestyle change on them. Things that people once relished start getting treated like toxic substances and after a while a lot of those people even stop enjoying those things altogether.

This is not just confined to food and lifestyle habits, a lot of other things like your income, your earning potential and maybe your ability to do things like you do today could expire too. Now that's just the ability part. It's also possible that your priorities change altogether and then that entire idea expires for you. Imagine if you weren't interested in money anymore. Imagine that 'prestige' as an idea didn't appeal to you anymore. Imagine you lost complete interest in entertainment, sex, good food, fast cars, travel, reading or anything else that mattered to you. Those aspects of your life will completely fade away. This is probably the most negative sounding article that I've ever written, but at the risk of adding to it, I just want to mention that there's always the possibility of people leaving us altogether. Though this is a term that I've only heard in India, there is probably a reason why they say that people "expire." The truth is that you never know when you might not be able to take the stairs anymore, when you have to stop eating wheat products for good, when you will stop being in love with someone, when you will have to stop travelling or when the last time that you might be seeing somebody is. You just never know.

Enjoy your life and everything in it while it lasts. Don't realise too late that you should have done what you wanted to. Sometimes you might not have the ability to do them anymore, and sometimes you might not even want to do them anymore.

Carpe Diem.

THEN WHAT MAKES LIFE WORTHWHILE

A SNAPSHOT

The start of this chapter is a look at how the typical approach of reading to find answers to questions like "What makes life worthwhile?" don't always work. A lot of us look at what's on the surface and say, "That's why I want to be alive," "That's what I love about life" and "That's why life's worth living." This chapter is about looking beyond the obvious. Most of us anyway keep resetting our goalposts of achievement and happiness. What makes life worth living today might not be what makes it worth living a few years or even a few months from now. I've discussed here some things that have a much longer shelf life, as areas to invest your time and energy in, for life. As the lyrics of the Pink Floyd song *Free Four*[12] go...

The memories of a man in his old age

Are the deeds of a man in his prime.

You shuffle in gloom of the sickroom

And talk to yourself as you die.

Life is a short, warm moment

And death is a long, cold rest.

You get your chance to try in the twinkling of an eye:

Eighty years, with luck, or even less.

Since our time on this planet is limited, it's worth spending it only on the most important things. A big part of wellbeing is about living a good life. This obviously calls for certain things to do, some things to watch out for and certainly building and keeping the right perspective. I talk here about what's worth pursuing, what's a good way of being and how not to go overboard with either.

WHY A LOT OF SELF-HELP BOOKS HARDLY HELP

Having been a corporate trainer and organisational development consultant for many years now, I have ended up reading a lot of books on self-development. A lot of times because of my own interest and I must confess, a few times also under the pressure of necessity. To deliver a particular kind of workshop for a specific client.

There are tonnes of books out there that focus merely on spreading knowledge. Well, if it's just about spreading knowledge, I don't think I've come across any book that doesn't meet the mark. Such books are necessary, and they have their own significance. A world atlas is a superb example. You don't need to build any particular skill or behaviour to know where the different countries of the world are located in relation to the others. It's ridiculous and impractical to start learning where the different countries are located through a hands-on and experiential means of visiting them for real. The issue is that a lot of people pick up self-help books with the hope of building a new competence or developing a new ability. Eventually, what ends up happening most of the time is that they gain knowledge about that area in terms of how important it is, why it is important, what are the different dimensions of it, even techniques used by people who are the icons of possessing and demonstrating that competence, and the story ends there. You finish the book, and you haven't become any more competent than before you started it. A good self-help book ought to be telling you how exactly to build a new skill or develop a new behaviour especially in terms of what exactly to do.

I've read several books that I obviously wouldn't want to name, but books that are over 200 pages, where there isn't a single thing that you can do. Developing a new ability is all about knowing what to do differently and how to practice that time and again till it becomes a skill. Likewise, knowing what to do and how to develop the willingness to do it repeatedly till it becomes a demonstrable behaviour. Of course, I don't want to talk as if all the books out there are full of junk and don't help you develop any ability whatsoever. No. There are a lot of wonderful books out there that clearly highlight what someone must do to get better or develop a new ability. One that lingers in my mind is B.K.S. Iyengar's book, *Light on Yoga*[13].

B.K.S. Iyengar[14] died in the year 2015, but he was one of the leading experts in the world on yoga. He had been teaching yoga since 1936 and had given demonstrations throughout the world. *Light on Yoga* is a book that tells you about various dimensions of yoga both as a practice and as a way of life. It's a book loaded with specific behaviours. It specifically tells you **what to do**. It's a classic book on yoga that clearly describes in a step-by-step manner how to practice various asanas or postures in yoga. Here's a breakup of what's written on the opening page of the book.

The skill – "… Practical and extensively illustrated, it describes over 200 postures (asanas and bandhas) and fourteen breathing exercises (pranayamas) in detail. The 600 photographs, placed in the relevant parts of the text, enable the reader to practice a posture without a teacher."

Knowledge – "There is a summary of the meaning of Yoga, and the nadis, chakras and kundalini are also considered…"

Behaviour – "…an appendix directs the reader to specific exercises for a wide variety of ailments and for the serious student, there is a long yoga course of over 300 weeks…"

There are several wonderful books out there on topics ranging from stress management to leadership to public speaking to solving crosswords that knock the nail on the head. That means they tell you for the most part what exactly you need to do to get better. On the contrary, there are loads of books that make ridiculous statements throughout that leave readers absolutely clueless about what they need to do. Here are some actual ones that I've picked out from books, magazine articles and blogs.

1. Focus on your strengths
2. Take ownership
3. Be more confident
4. Be proactive instead of reactive
5. Lead by example
6. Start communicating clearly
7. Be motivated
8. Trust yourself
9. Don't regret thinking about the past
10. Set clear goals and work on achieving them

11. Find your passion and make it your vocation
12. Always have a healthy self-esteem
13. Work hard
14. Be more dedicated towards your priorities
15. Relax
16. Don't worry
17. Think out of the box
18. Learn from your failures
19. Think positively or always look on the brighter side
20. Have a clear purpose in life

Telling someone to be confident tells them nothing about any specific behaviour. About what exactly they need to do the next time around when they want to be confident. The same is true of telling someone to relax, work hard, be motivated or trust others or for that matter trust in themselves.

Now this is just one half of the problem with respect to why some self-help books don't work. The other half and the more critical and heavier half of the problem, in my view, is that a great number of self-help books (and by that I mean a far greater number than the ones that don't tell you exactly what to do) actually don't help you help yourself. In fact, several books end up making you not just feel but become worse than you initially were.

What is striking to me is the fact that many of the self-help books and videos and even trainers, coaches and self-development programmes focus on faking it rather than being it. Participants sometimes ask me at the start of some of my public speaking and presentation workshops if at the end of the workshop they will be able to look more confident, seem relaxed while presenting and come across as effective presenters. I often have to clarify to them that my workshops are not about looking and acting like. The best way to look confident is to first be confident and then just look normal. The best way to look relaxed is to actually be relaxed. No one ever comes across as an effective presenter until he or she is truly an effective presenter. While this phenomenon of 'acting like' is really pronounced in the self-help industry that focuses on sales and selling, it is prevalent in all dimensions of self-help.

You have techniques to build rapport with your client, techniques to close deals, objection-handling techniques, tips to negotiate better, interest-creating remarks, FAB statements and the list goes on. In the long run, nothing works better than actually having rapport and trust with a client, creating a product that is truly beneficial and giving the client the best value for his money. What many don't realise is that it hardly helps to act like someone you are not. Working on or training yourself to look successful, appear competent or act happy actually takes you further away from actually being successful, competent and experiencing true happiness. It's about what's inside rather than what's merely on the surface. It's about actually transforming rather than trying to look different from the outside. It's about internal cures and being at peace with yourself rather than cosmetic surgeries and living the life of a wannabe.

The next time you plan to buy a book that is supposed to help you get better, beyond just gathering more ideas. Flip through its pages and look at how much of the book focuses on specific things to do. Does it tell you to sit down on a chair, keep your spine erect, close your eyes gently and take a deep breath? Or does it just say "You must relax"? You are better off using a book that outlines specific behaviours clearly to you. A word of caution is to not expect details of specific behaviours to practice on each and every page or in each chapter. Then you'll end up buying nothing.

LOOKING BEYOND THE OBVIOUS

I'd like to use the Alpha Male as a metaphor for how people might sometimes see just what's on the surface of life and not beyond. Things that meet the eye and not what underlies the entire phenomenon. I'm in no way supportive of people who are alpha males, nor do I have anything against them. I feel neutral and don't care one way or the other. But what interests me is the stereotype that surrounds the alpha male in many parts of the world. That, I think, is worth examining, both as a way to understand some of the stereotypes that surround life itself and the way we try to live it.

The misconceptions about the concept of the alpha male range from people seeing it as the ultimate acknowledgement of a man's virility to feeling the need to be aggressive or flirt with women. Saying that being an alpha male is just about being physically fit, behaviourally aggressive or smooth with women is like reducing Osho's entire range of ideas and philosophies merely to what he said about sex. So what else makes an alpha male?

First of all, an alpha male is not a bully. He is not out there to get other people or put others down. On the contrary, he is someone who lifts people up and brings out the best in them. That's precisely what makes him stand out and shine in a group. Quite like the lion that is seen as the king of the jungle and yet doesn't kill his prey for cheap thrills. But when a lion is hungry or needs to attack, he knows exactly what to do. Even the alpha male attacks only under the pressure of necessity, and when he does, size doesn't matter. His energy in a fight is immense and mostly drawn from within rather than through practice or technique.

Second, the alpha male is not stuck up. He is a flexible beast. He accepts mistakes, takes ownership and adapts quickly. He realises that negative feedback or differences in opinion are not a personal insult to his manhood or to himself as a human being. He is calm, composed and has a striking sense of poise even when things are not going his way. This comes from his quality of not blaming others, taking responsibility for who he is and his remarkable optimism in learning, growing and becoming a better person.

Another brilliant quality the alpha male possesses is being comfortable with being exactly who he is. He doesn't suck up to anybody in the face of hierarchical superiority, greater public image or under social pressure. He speaks his mind out, doesn't mince words and shoots bullets of honesty through his language and actions. This ability to express himself with ease makes him a fascinating leader, beyond just good decision making or being at the helm of affairs in any setup.

Finally, one more defining factor of an alpha male is that he is passionate about life. He sees a clear purpose to his existence and as a result, finds more meaning in his work, his actions and his life as a whole. He clearly stands for certain things, and that gives him a sense of style and charisma that is truly his and not one prescribed by others.

An alpha male doesn't need to be young. You can be an alpha male at any age, and there could be several other factors that define an alpha male to a slightly lesser degree than the ones described above. But for the most part, he is seen as someone who can walk into a room, fill it with his presence, exposing himself completely with uncrossed hands, direct eye contact and engaging others through his entertaining stories and his sense of humour. In a world where political correctness reigns supreme, the alpha male will continue to express himself and yet there is one thing that he never does. He never tries to be an alpha male. He stays who he is, and the fact that he's an alpha male is just incidental.

That's also exactly what happens in life. People sometimes get bogged down by the obvious and don't see beyond it. Getting overwhelmed by the pursuit of material possessions and momentary highs cause some of them to miss the larger point of living and loving life. Like the alpha male, the really happy people are not trying hard to be happy. That's just who they are.

A QUICK WAY TO TAME YOUR EGO

For the sake of this piece, I'm not referring to ego merely as the consciousness of your identity or the "I" as Freud called it. I'm referring to the inflated feeling of pride that some of us sometimes feel in our superiority over others. Taming your ego is not about putting an end to the ego and killing it altogether. This causes a person to miss out even on the good aspects of having a healthy respect for their identity. My focus is to ensure that you aren't being controlled by your ego to a point where it constantly influences your behaviour, and you have no way out. As Friedrich Nietzsche put it, "Whenever I climb I am followed by a dog called 'Ego.'"

Begin by thinking about a situation when you behaved in a certain way because of your ego. Maybe you screamed at someone, stopped being in touch with someone, walked out of a restaurant, lied about something or even drove rashly. Now think about what your ultimate goal was in that situation. Imagine you walked into a restaurant to have dinner, ordered your food, but walked out before it arrived because you weren't happy with the waiter's service. Your specific behaviour in that situation was to walk out of the restaurant before your food arrived. Your ultimate goal in that situation was to actually eat a good dinner. Then ask yourself if your behaviour supported your ultimate goal. If yes, then great.

On the contrary, if you walked out because your ego had filled you with a sense of entitlement, that you need to be served as soon as you walk into a restaurant, then the only thing you achieved was staying hungry a little longer or even skipping dinner. In which case, you ended up doing something because of your ego that took you further away from your ultimate goal of wanting to enjoy a good dinner. Every time you notice that you've done something because of your ego, that's taken you away from your ultimate goal or what you actually wanted to have, then you better rethink that behaviour. The final step is to do something different or adopt a new behaviour the next time around. Or even do something right now that will help you undo the damage caused by your past ego-driven behaviour. If you screamed at a friend and that severed your relationship, and your real goal was to retain that person as a friend, then maybe you should swallow your pride, call up and apologise. The next time you're at a restaurant and the food is a few minutes late, realise that it's you who needs dinner and not the waiter. So stay put or request the waiter again to speed up. Call the management and give them some feedback if you like.

People I've suggested this to started doing it for several instances from their lives where their ego caused them to act or behave in a certain way. Eventually, this got them to act differently the next time a similar situation arose. Do this, and in due course, you'll start doing the right thing in different situations out of instinct rather than being controlled by your ego.

LIFE IS A PURSUIT
OF EXCELLENCE

We're all trying to get better in life in some aspect all the time. We're on a continuous pursuit of excellence. When I look around, I see people either trying to make more money, get healthier, run faster, become more competent in some area at work, become better parents, get promoted, find more leisure time, pursue higher spiritual goals and so on. It doesn't matter what you're trying to do; the point is that you're always trying to pursue excellence of some kind. Even those who are trying to quit their jobs and focus on a hobby are trying to pursue excellence in living a balanced life. One of the best ways to do this is to study other people who you think have achieved excellence and apply the lessons you learn into your own life. I'd like to first do this for you with someone I consider to be excellent. That should give you a sense of how to do it yourself later to someone who you think has succeeded in his or her pursuit of excellence.

The person who I am about to describe here is the writer Robert M. Pirsig[15]. He has achieved excellence both in terms of his writing as well as in terms of his understanding of what he writes about. He died in April 2017 but has left behind strong clues and inputs for an excellent life.

So, do I think he's excellent?

Yes, of course.

The next question is, "Why do I think he's excellent?"

He's excellent as a writer because his two books *Zen and the Art of Motorcycle Maintenance*[16] and *Lila*[17] are indicators of how something so complex and yet so fundamental can be put across in writing in a way that is not just understandable but also insightful and inspiring. It might be somewhat easier to write fiction because there is a storyline, there are characters, there is the climax, suspense and the possibility of creating things that don't exist just to keep the reader engrossed. In my view, the true mettle of a writer really comes out when none of those things exist and yet the writing is made interesting. To beat that, Pirsig also talks about ideas that are heavy, penetrating them to their depths and clarifying debatable concepts to the reader through the book. That, to me, is an excellent writer.

The lesson that I gather here about excellence is to make the complex understandable and to simplify things overall. Now how do I use this in my life and my own pursuit of excellence?

Why else do I think he's excellent?

The other reason that I consider Robert Pirsig to be excellent is because of what he writes about. The taglines of his two books really explain that. *Zen and the Art of Motorcycle Maintenance: An Inquiry into Values* and *Lila: An Inquiry into Morals*. To think of it, it all started when he was a teacher, and one of his colleagues casually made a statement to him on campus, "I hope you are teaching quality to your students." Robert Pirsig's interest in quality and journey into understanding it better starts there. Then he goes so deep into it that he actually ends up writing two books about it. The idea of a person wanting to make sure that he is earnestly teaching quality to his students, having the commitment to go so deep into something and creating a body of knowledge around it is just incredible. This, to me, is not just a pursuit of excellence but a symbol of excellence in and of itself.

The lesson that I gather here about excellence is to dig deeper into whatever you are pursuing in life rather than skim the surface. So, again, I ask myself, "How do I use this in my life and my own pursuit of excellence?"

The next step is to look at what this person said. Both in terms of his ideas as well as what he stood for.

Robert Pirsig's work has a lot to do with the whole idea of quality. I think he was to a large extent talking about living a good life and appreciating the good things in it. He just didn't call it that. He called it quality. While the book *Zen and the Art of Motorcycle Maintenance* actually suggests how riding a motorcycle can be a mindful and meditative experience, some of his quotes[18] below sum up the dimensions of a high-quality life that he's touched upon.

"The only Zen you can find on the tops of mountains is the Zen you bring up there."

"Quality is a direct experience independent of and prior to intellectual abstractions."

"To live only for some future goal is shallow. It's the sides of the mountain that sustain life, not the top."

"The Buddha resides as comfortably in the circuits of a digital computer or the gears of a cycle transmission as he does at the top of a mountain."

"The funny thing about insane people is that it is kind of the opposite of being a celebrity. Nobody envies you."

"It is a puzzling thing. The truth knocks on the door and you say, 'Go away, I'm looking for the truth,' and so it goes away. Puzzling."

"The study of the art of motorcycle maintenance is really a miniature study of the art of rationality itself. Working on a motorcycle, working well, caring, is to become part of a process, to achieve an inner peace of mind. The motorcycle is primarily a mental phenomenon."

Now, what do I gather from the above ideas and expressions and how can I demonstrate and practice them in my own life?

One of the important lessons to derive from this quick analysis of someone who I think is excellent, is to identify clues and inputs from their lives in terms of what they did, how they did it, what they said and believed in. Then absorb those lessons and qualities into your own life by following their insights and demonstrating them.

Remember, Robert Pirsig here is just an example. You should only do this for someone who YOU think has been successful in their pursuit of excellence.

WHO IS THE ONE PERSON WHO MATTERS THE MOST TO YOU?

The role of the one person who matters the most to you could start well before you are born. To the unborn child, the mother could clearly be the most important person, as everything from the child's nutrition to other bodily functions depend on her. As we all go through life, we meet, interact and sometimes live with different people. Though all these people fit different roles in our lives, there is always that one person who clearly matters the most to each of us at any given point.

This is a sort of construct that lies in the inner realms of your mind and could remain there forever unless, God forbid, you are in a hostage situation or a crazy reality show where you might have to disclose it. Of course, there are some parents who put children through the dilemma of having to choose their favourite between the two parents, sometimes casually, by verbally asking the child to do so and sometimes more seriously, through action as a result of an unavoidable separation or divorce. In any case, this one person who matters the most in your life could change, and on many occasions, several times during the lifespan of one individual. The person who mattered the most to you as a child, like your mother or father might mostly not even be around in the October, November and December of your life and this role could be taken up by your spouse, son, daughter or even a home nurse or caretaker. Between these two extremes of childhood and old age, you might have different people who matter to you the most at different points, for several reasons.

Changing Roles

If the most prominent role you play in life is that of a father, the person who matters the most could be your child or one of your children who you feel needs you more. If the biggest role you play is that of a wife, then the person who matters the most to you is likely to be your husband. With changes in the most significant role that you play in life, that one person who matters the most could keep changing.

Changing Emotions

We spend most of our lives chasing different emotions. These emotions could be love, happiness, pride, security, satisfaction, peace, etc. At any given point, there is one emotion that overshadows the rest of them and that hugely determines who the one person who matters the most in your life could be at that point. If you're chasing security, that one person could be the one who gives you that security. If you are chasing love, that one person might be the one who gives you the love you crave for.

Changing Situations

Even those who believed that they would never be able to live without that one person who mattered the most in their lives have been proved wrong and in certain cases, several times over. People fall out of love, people change priorities in life, people change organisations, careers and countries. Sometimes people even die and leave us for good. Any of these could cause you to change in your mind the one person who matters the most. You might hang on to the memories of the person who left you or try to bridge the gap between distance and geography by staying in touch, but the void eventually gets filled by another person.

While these were more stable scenarios and might only change over longer periods of time, at a micro level, the person who matters the most to you could change in several ways.

Seeking Approval

In life, the person whose approval you seek could change from time to time. If you've accomplished something great, that moment might not be complete for you till you let that special person know and gain their acknowledgement or appreciation. This person could be a sweetheart, a superior, a parent, a mentor or even an arch-rival. For some, this person might also vanish altogether especially when they overcome their concern about public opinion or social approval. When they move into a state of doing things for their satisfaction and purely because they want to, than for someone else.

Finding Solutions

People are faced with various kinds of difficulties and challenges at different points in life. Someone who is bankrupt and struggling to come out of it might see the person who can bail them out as the one who matters to them the most at that moment. A person battling a terminal illness will see anyone who can provide a miraculous treatment and cure as the person who matters the most for that time.

Taking Things for Granted

There is something about the threat of losing a person that makes that person the most important person at that point in time. It's quite common in organisations that an employee is overloaded, not compensated adequately and completely taken for granted. This goes on until the employee finally gets sick and tired of working there and decides to quit. At this point, he or she becomes the person who matters the most and many others in the organisation are trying to make the employee feel good and hold the person back. A similar phenomenon occurs in relationships where a couple is together for several years or sometimes just months and gradually and often without their knowledge, start taking each other for granted. Typically one of them is more on the receiving end of the unreasonable behaviour and lack of care or love from the other in spite of repeated reminders. At some point, the victim can take it no more and pulls the plug on the relationship; and when that happens, he or she becomes the all-important person in the world for the other.

The other person could go out of their way and do things that he or she has never done before to fix the relationship and get their partner back.

Put Yourself First

In almost all the above cases, the one person who matters the most in your life has been someone else. There's always the option of considering yourself to be that one person. While some might see this as being self-absorbed or even selfish, I think it's absolutely normal and even desirable to make yourself the one person who matters the most in your life. People end up doing all sorts of things like moving to a new city or country, taking up or quitting a job, developing new behaviours or stopping old ones and sometimes even parting with loved ones for the sake of the person who matters the most to them. This being the case, it makes perfect sense to put yourself at the centre of your universe. More importantly, whether it means being there for the person who you love the most in this world or experiencing sweet revenge by getting back at your worst enemy, your presence is indispensable. All the needs of every single person who matters to you can be met only if you're around. If you're not, the link between yourself and the outer world won't be established. Now isn't that obvious.

In his work *Politics*[19], Aristotle says, "Man is by nature a social animal; an individual who is unsocial naturally and not accidentally is either beneath our notice or more than human. Society is something that precedes the individual. Anyone who either cannot lead the common life or is so self-sufficient as not to need to and therefore does not partake of society, is either a beast or a god."

In my view, making yourself the person who matters the most to you is in no way more superior to having someone else fulfil that role. Selflessness and altruism are perspectives just like self-centricity and egoism. They are both different and valid in their own right.

IF YOU HAVE AN OPTION – CHOOSE TO BE NICE

I was once on an Air France flight to Spain, and among other things, one thing that I constantly notice because of my interest in human behaviour is the way the cabin crew interact with the guests as well as with each other. Out of the three stewards and four stewardesses, one gentleman really stood out from the others. He was a cut above the rest in terms of both the quality of his service as well as his aura and the energy that he spread around him. His name was Jon Paul (I asked him later). As I sat there with the constant hum of the aircraft in the background, wondering what made this man exceptional, it suddenly struck me that it wasn't that he was more competent as a steward or he knew the dishes on the menu any better or even that he was the lead flight attendant. He was just nicer. To all his colleagues as well as to all the guests onboard.

This is the single most important quality that will help you leverage all the other strengths that you have. It's also one that is greatly overlooked in the entire field of self-development, in a world of achievement orientation and 'get what you want' thinking.

I remember having a conversation a while ago with a group of veteran advertising professionals. They spoke about a time in the field of advertising when a really creative person could pretty much do what he or she felt like and get away with it. Their high score on the creativity scale, sort of compensated for their other tantrums. But in today's advertising industry, along with being creative, you also have to be nice. While I agree with the idea of niceness playing a critical role, I certainly don't think that it's a recent feature in our lives.

Human beings are inherently attracted to niceness. We've always been. We'd rather spend time with people who are nice to us especially since most human beings anyway, are in their nicest behaviour when they are in a good mood and when things are going well for them. I've met a few extremely competent people in my career who've struggled to grow, purely because their competence was shrouded by rudeness or outright arrogance. Now I'm not suggesting that you use niceness as a strategy, because that seems to be the sad mantra of the 21st century – reducing every great human quality into a formula for success. On the contrary, there's a whole lot of literature out there that opposes niceness, where phrases like "The nice guys finish last" and "Nice is just a place in France" have become popular punch lines.

I don't encourage anyone to be nice because they are going to get a better job, close more deals or find love. That thinking is fundamentally flawed and will never be nice. There is real charm in being nice for niceness's sake, and that in itself is the symbol of a better life. That is exactly what even the nice steward Jon Paul told me after the flight landed in Barcelona, and I asked him what makes him be so nice to everyone even when no one's watching. He had just two simple things to say: "It's nicer to be nice" and "Being nice also makes you feel nicer."

ARE YOU SUFFERING FROM 21ST CENTURY COMPASSION FATIGUE?

Actual Compassion Fatigue[20] was a term first referred to in a U.S. document on immigration policy in the early 1980s. It refers to the progressive fading away of compassion among individuals who need to express high levels of compassion as a result of the work they do or because of the life situations they are in.

In my view, the legitimate version of compassion fatigue that results from a continuous exposure to painful situations is clearly understandable. For example, taking care of a bedridden family member for a prolonged period of time, going through a complicated and traumatic divorce that is spread over years or working a job that involves exposure to people in some sort of pain or trauma. But today, people seem to be victims of compassion fatigue even when there's nothing in particular to be fatigued about. I'm more interested in talking about the 21st century variant of compassion fatigue, where it's not just trauma or pain but various other emotions that people are fatigued towards. There's an overload of exposure today towards certain dimensions of life and this, in turn, leads to people becoming numb to what an acceptable dose of the related emotions might be.

Though leading bodies in the world, like the World Health Organisation and the American Psychiatric Association are yet to accept compassion fatigue as an actual diagnosis, there's simply no debate about a gradual numbing effect that occurs to people's reactions and perceptions to certain things due to overexposure. Versions of compassion fatigue, in my view, are present in several walks of life, even if you're not in a job that requires taking care of others or showing compassion. The phenomena of eating and drinking out regularly, divorces, depression, traffic jams or long commutes, and several other negative hallmarks of big cities have gone up so much that you might well be partaking in the madness and not realising it.

In the corporate world, the incessant cribbing that I often hear from people who I meet almost makes job dissatisfaction a given. Monday morning blues and TGIF are accepted norms in most parts of the world. To the extent that if you don't complain about your job, you might stick out like a sore thumb in some organisations.

Another roaring example is social media. With the ever-increasing popularity of Facebook, Twitter, Whatsapp and Snapchat, a segment of people are simply too used to sharing every single detail about themselves with the rest of the world. As a result, the sharing quotient of most social media users in the world has gone through the roof. More importantly, there's this constant pressure of having to portray a good life as if your existing life and what you have is seriously flawed.

The great danger of a continuous exposure to excesses is that it warps your sense of what's acceptable and what you actually feel like. Don't get so used to broadcasting your life that privacy means nothing to you anymore. Don't chase your financial dreams so hard that you're unable to enjoy the money you already have. Don't be so obsessed with trying to look better that you stop appreciating your personality and charm. As the Chicago Tribune columnist Mary Schmich put it, "Enjoy the power and beauty of your youth. Oh, never mind. You will not understand the power and beauty of your youth until they've faded. But trust me, in twenty years, you'll look back at photos of yourself and recall in a way you can't grasp now how much possibility lay before you and how fabulous you really looked. You are not as fat as you imagine."

Most importantly, don't be so caught up in trying to live a successful life that you forget to live a happy one.

FAILURE IS NOT THE OPPOSITE OF SUCCESS

In an interview I read, Arianna Huffington, the co-founder and editor-in-chief of The Huffington Post said, "My mother used to say failure is not the opposite of success, it's a stepping-stone to success." When I first heard that sentence, I couldn't help thinking how clichéd the second part of that sentence sounded. But on playing it and replaying it in my head, that old cliché made new sense to me. Also because it was Arianna Huffington, who is herself a drum major for promoting wellbeing, I started thinking of this in the light of health and wellbeing too.

Quite a few people look at health and wellbeing in terms of zeroes or ones, black or white, healthy or unhealthy, happy or unhappy, etc. The point is that such people see the ideal state to be a success and everything else to be failures. Paunch versus six-pack, fat versus slim, tired versus energetic, drowsy versus alert, flabby versus muscular, weak versus strong, depressed versus elated, anxious versus relaxed and many more. So having a six-pack is seen as a success and anything else is seen as a failure, or being relaxed is viewed as a success and anything less than that is viewed as a failure. In reality, a pot belly and a six-pack are two ends of the same spectrum, just like anxious and relaxed are.

When you start looking at health and wellbeing in this way, you realise that tired, drowsy, flabby, weak, depressed, etc., are just points on different continua that let you know exactly where you are. Contemporary ideas in self-development and personal growth strongly emphasise this.

- There is no failure, only feedback.
- If what you're doing isn't working, do something else. Anything else.
- Doing the same things and expecting different results is the definition of insanity.

The above are just three out of several popular adages that support the "Failure is not the opposite of success" idea. Even in the sphere of wellbeing, failure is just a state where you've stopped trying. Anything else is a success.

Of course, I don't want to sound as if failure is the most comfortable spot to be in. It's not. That's exactly why it's the place where you get maximum feedback from. It is from this point that it could be most difficult to take action. Even physically, it could be more difficult for an obese person to do 100 push-ups than it might be for someone who is slim and fit. Consider the following scenarios.

- If your exercise plan or diet has not helped you get into the desired fitness level, don't back out. Do something else. Anything else. Analyse what could have gone wrong with that particular diet or exercise plan, make changes and try it again or in the worst case, at least move on to another diet or fitness plan.
- Imagine you're a long distance runner and you've steadily been clocking better finishing times

marathon after marathon for the first five marathons. Then suddenly, for the next two marathons, your finishing time has dropped drastically. That's no reason to stop running altogether. Every running enthusiast knows that. These are opportunities to review your practice sessions, diet, the terrain of the run, the temperature, what you kept telling yourself, etc. Then make the required changes and run the next marathon.

❖ In the course of our lives, there are likely to be times when we land up with some major illnesses like cancer, heart disease, rheumatoid arthritis, diabetes, etc. When this happens, there are many who see the situation as "Earlier I was healthy and now I am sick." Period. Once again, it's not sick versus healthy. You are better off telling yourself, "Earlier I was very healthy, and now I am less healthy," and then doing what you need to do to improve your health. Drink more water, eat healthier, get more rest, sleep a little longer, start exercising or take the right medication regularly. In any case, sitting back and doing nothing about it isn't going to help much.

So the title of this article is obviously not meant to be a lesson in English grammar but a new approach to wellbeing and life in general.

THE BEHAVIOURAL SIDE OF WELLBEING

A SNAPSHOT

It's not that we're not interested in reaching a greater state of wellbeing; it's not that we aren't capable or lack the ability. The challenges that I hear most people I coach or train mention is that they're either too busy or are just unable to adopt and practice the very things that they know would make them feel good. A lot of us are way too busy to live the life we actually deserve and struggle with changing the way we do things.

Having referred to behaviour so many times until this point in this book, this chapter is where I say a bit about it. To me, Behaviour is best defined as "anything you do." You will get a glimpse in this chapter of how, in the end, irrespective of what you're trying to achieve in the realm of wellbeing or otherwise, developing desired behaviours is at the heart of it all. You'll also see why a lot us do the things that we do and what steps might help you do things differently. Including practical ways to change existing behaviours and develop new ones. I've been working in the field of people development with corporates and individuals for over fifteen years now. In all this time, there's absolutely nothing that I've come across that involves people getting different or better results without them changing their behaviours. So if you want to read just one chapter of this book and read no more, then this chapter should be it.

WELLNESS BEHAVIOURS PRECEDE WELLBEING

Some years ago, I was driving back home early in the morning on the first of January, having slept over at a friend's place after the New Year's party. I was on a long and winding stretch of road in my city, and I was amazed at the number of people I saw who were either running, jogging or walking. I told myself, "Wow! The city is, in fact, getting fitter." Roughly a month later, I was on that same stretch at around the same time, driving to a hotel for a training programme. The number of people I saw had easily dropped to one-tenth of what it was on the first of January. The people who are walking or running in the morning past January are likely to be the ones who were doing it even in December the previous year. A New Year's resolution can only take you that far. A lot of folks consider physical wellness as a big part of wellbeing. But what's more crucial than registering for a fitness programme is to develop the right habits or what I call "Wellness Behaviours." A large financial investment made towards a fitness programme might create a momentary sense of commitment, but this rarely leads to long-term endurance.

Use some of these tips instead, as they've helped a lot of my corporate clients develop Wellness Behaviours and reach a better state of wellbeing over time.

Dress Rehearsal

If your fitness programme is a kick-boxing class at 6 a.m. in the morning, first practice waking up at 5:30 a.m. and getting completely ready, including wearing your kick-boxing gear. You will do everything except the actual class. If you can do this for twenty-one days, it means you are ready to register for the class. You might see this as a horrendous waste of time, but this is the most critical part where you're building new behaviour. There's a reason why even the best performers in the world do a dress rehearsal. The idea is to practice exactly the steps where you might goof up later. In this case, waking up early and getting ready to go for your class.

Simplification

For many, getting ready to go to the gym is one activity. Getting to the gym is another activity. Working out at the gym is yet another activity and getting back home is one more activity. Do what it takes to simplify this. Sign up at the gym closest to home, invest in home-fitness equipment or even go to bed in your workout clothes if possible. It helps to reduce the number of steps in the process of getting fit and reduce the related complexity. You are more likely to put things away when they are complex.

Just Do It

When it is time for you to work out, don't stop to think, just do it. The moment you start thinking, a part of your brain comes up with justifications and will give you a range of reasons to not go through the strain of a workout or a difficult drive to the gym. The same applies when your alarm goes off in the morning. Don't think. Just get out of bed and get started. Likewise, if you plan to go for a walk after you get back home from work. Then get back home, change and get going. Don't tell yourself, "Well, I'll just sit on the couch, catch just one episode of *Friends* and then head for my walk." Because before you know it, you could be four episodes and three beers down, wanting to just get dinner and hit the bed.

Attack When the Going Gets Tough

There are days when it's raining, when you have a mild headache, when you've hardly slept the previous night because of an important presentation or your child was ill. By ensuring that you work out even on such days, you give your brain two powerful messages. First, "Not working out is not an option" and second, "Your willpower will overshadow your brain's justifications for not working out." With repetition, your brain realises that the only option is to workout. Over time, it even stops looking at or evaluating other options.

The Last Resort – Have Fewer Rules

As a means to adapt to the demands of reality, allow yourself some flexibility.

- ❖ Working out any five days of the week.
- ❖ Working out at any time of the day.
- ❖ If the fitness centre is shut, do some other kind of workout.
- ❖ If your only pair of running shoes got stolen, take a walk in your floaters.
- ❖ If your gym instructor is under the weather, work out alone, etc.

As a long-term strategy to your wellbeing, acquire and grow the right behaviours. This helps you get the best out of life, not just with respect to a fitness programme, but also for anything you want to achieve.

FIVE BASIC TRUTHS ABOUT YOUR BEHAVIOUR

Knowing what your behaviour is, is the starting point of managing it better. Many conventional definitions of behaviour spoke about it being a response to some sort of stimulus, being a range of actions or mannerisms of a being or system and some even related behaviour to the natural way of doing things. I think those are all great ways to look at behaviour. Yet, knowing what it is might just be a starting point. It's important to see some obvious and useful truths about your behaviour in order to help you use it as an instrument for wellbeing.

Behaviour Is What You Do

One of the best definitions that I've come across in recent times is – A behaviour is anything you do. If you stand erect, that's a behaviour. If you slouch when you sit down, that's a behaviour; if you brush your teeth every morning, that's a behaviour. The point is that behaviour is not just confined to anything you do physically; it also refers to anything you do mentally. If you say, "Oh no! Not again!" to yourself mentally whenever you face a difficulty, that's a behaviour. If you go inward or get lost in thought when someone's talking to you, that's a behaviour too.

Each Behaviour Gets Easier with Practice

This means a couple of things. If you do something once, it is easy to do it again. If you smoke once, it is easy to smoke again. If you fast once, it is easy to fast again. If you do something with a person once, it is easy to repeat that behaviour with that person again. If you tell someone a secret and build trust once, you are likely to share more with that person. Also, your behaviour could influence the behaviour of the people around you and vice versa. For instance, if you hang out with a group of biking enthusiasts, your own alignment towards biking is likely to increase.

Your Behaviour Is the Window to Your Attitude

Your attitude is a mental appraising statement about the world around you. For the most part, nobody gets to see what's running through your head. Yet, the moment you behave, people get a glimpse into your attitude. All the world sees is your behaviour, and different people might interpret your behaviour differently based on their own attitudes, backgrounds and baggage.

You Can Choose Your Behaviour

One of the beautiful phenomena in life is that, with a little bit of effort, we can actually choose our behaviour. Even in an intense period of stress and uncertainty, you can choose to relax, provided you've practised the behaviour of relaxation often enough. Even when people around you are screaming in excitement, you can choose to be composed and grounded if you like. With each episode of demonstrating this behaviour, the easier it will get and the more likely you are to choose it again.

You Can Use Your Behaviour

The obvious next step once you've realised that you can choose your behaviour is to work towards using it wisely. You certainly don't want to choose the wrong behaviours and, in turn, ruin the quality of your life. There's an entire industry of personality and self-development that is based on the fact that you can choose your behaviour. It's almost impossible to change your attitude and at a deeper level your entire personality directly. The doorway to such deeper levels of transformation is your behaviour. By demonstrating a new and desirable behaviour even just once, you increase the possibility and ease of being able to repeat that behaviour. If repeated often enough, your outlook towards the situations where that behaviour is required will change (this is your new attitude). Several such attitude changes eventually change who you are as a person (this is your improved personality).

It all boils down to this, if you are at peace with who you are and want to remain there, just repeat your typical and routine behaviours. If you want to be a better person, choose better behaviours. If you want to be a happier person, choose happier behaviours. I think you know the rest.

LEVERAGING YOUR BEHAVIOUR FOR WELLBEING

Ask anyone who is in pursuit of wellbeing, their reason behind it. Or even just ask someone why they do anything at all in life. Just taking wellness as an example, before reading on, ask yourself why being in good health matters to you. Make a note of your responses. You're most likely to get responses that fall under one of these categories.

Pleasure-Seeking Responses

These are responses that suggest that the person wants to be healthy to in turn get to a number of other things. Typical responses of this sort include:

- ❖ To live longer
- ❖ To look good
- ❖ So that I can enjoy life
- ❖ It makes me happy, etc.

Pain-Avoiding Responses

These are responses that suggest that the person wants to be healthy and fit to in turn get away from a number of other things. Such responses include:

* To not get a heart attack
* To not be obese
* So that I'm not dependant on others
* So that I don't feel lousy about myself, etc.

Though "wellbeing or good health" as concepts are the same for everyone, people who fall under the above categories might approach wellness and life in general with entirely different mindsets.

The kinds of questions to ask yourself are:

* Do you work out to become slim or to lose weight?
* Do you work to become financially independent or to get out of debt?
* Do you want to stay healthy to be able to take vacations with your family and have fun for a long time to come or so that you don't leave your family in trouble if you die young?
* Do you want to stop worrying or do you want to be happy and content?
* Do you want to stop working late or do you want to start leaving early?

A logical answer for a lot of people is to say, "Both," and that is what leveraging behaviour is all about. It's about firing your enthusiasm and drive to practice certain behaviours for the pleasure of achievement and ensuring that you don't slow down or quit by reminding yourself of the pain that you might have to subject yourself to.

This idea could be traced back to the ancient Greek philosophers Democritus (460–370 B.C.) and

Aristippus (435–356 B.C.) who spoke of the pursuit of pleasure and the avoidance of pain as the key drivers of human behaviour.

Advertising is a field where this concept is particularly well understood. The next time you see an ad for a beauty product or for weight loss or hair loss with before and after pictures, remember that they're essentially saying, "This is what you don't want to be, and this is what you could be." In other words, they are encouraging you to avoid pain, being overweight, bald or in some cultures dark, and to start being fit, slim and with a head full of hair.

Now, look at your own responses to the question "Why good health matters to you?" and see if your responses include more pleasure-seeking or pain-avoiding elements. While one set of responses is not more superior than the other, what they do indicate is where your focus lies. An ideal approach is to use both pleasure-seeking and pain-avoiding elements to keep yourself in the middle path of the behaviour of your choice.

PLAYING THE PAIN-PLEASURE GAME RIGHT

We all tend to focus on different areas that are important to us in life. These could be health, wealth, happiness, love, security, peace of mind, social status, etc. Irrespective of what your focus areas are, pain and pleasure are like two ends of the spectrum.

Pleasure seekers tend to focus on what they want to achieve and where they want to head to. This approach is actively at work in people who say things like – I want a big car, I want a fancy mansion, I want to get rich, I want to go to the Himalayas this year, I want to be happy, etc. Pain avoiders tend to focus on what they don't want to have or where they don't want to be. This approach is actively at work in people who say things like – I don't want this small car anymore, I am tired of this tiny apartment, I don't want to remain poor and keep struggling to pay my bills, I don't want to go to a cold place, I don't want to be sad anymore, etc. While both these approaches are different, they're also versions of each other. You will rarely find a person whose approach is purely pleasure-seeking or purely pain-avoiding, and in reality, most people function from both these approaches to some degree or another. Having said that, it's also fair to say that there are many individuals for whom one approach completely overshadows the other.

Everyone knows that you tend to materialise and bring into your physical reality what you think of and visualise. This idea has been so popularised over the years that you've surely heard statements that prescribe it like:

"What you see is what you get."

"Thoughts become things. So choose them wisely."

"You will step into the life you visualise."

Using the pleasure-seeking approach is a great way to get exactly what you want in life. You will live your ideal life if you first start seeing that ideal life in your mind and start focusing on it rather than focusing on the kind of life you don't want. If you want to get a master's degree or a Ph.D., then set clear goals and work towards them rather than figuring out ways to live with your undergraduate degree. You are more likely to have peace of mind by figuring out ways to create that peace of mind for yourself as opposed to focusing on the zillion activities in your life that are keeping you tensed and worried.

The pain-avoiding approach is a great way to jolt yourself out of a state of unnecessary complacency or carelessness. Imagine if you were an obese person who's been working out for a year and have slowed down now since you've lost a lot of weight, you can regain momentum by briefly reminding yourself of your previous obese state and how you could fall back into it if not cautious.

Interestingly, the approach you use changes the way you experience life, the speed at which you achieve results as well as the kind of results you achieve. While one approach is not better than the other, they are both significant in their own sweet ways. Pain, after all, is not always a bad thing. Let the pain chase you in the direction of your dreams while the pleasure draws you into its sweetness.

REPRODUCING EXCELLENCE

When Arnold Schwarzenegger was asked in an interview about how he went on to become a successful Hollywood star, he rattled off a remarkably simple answer. He said something that really highlighted the essence of what most people are trying to do while they're pursuing wellbeing.

There is an entire field called NLP[21]. It stands for Neuro-Linguistic Programming, and it's been a bit of a buzzword for the past couple of decades. Putting it simply, NLP is a way of achieving the outcomes you want by using thought, language and behaviour appropriately. Meaning, it is a way to create and reproduce excellence by coding some of the elements and principles of excellence. What NLP says is that if someone can do something well, you can reproduce that. More importantly, if you can do something well, then you can reproduce that in other areas of your life too. This essentially means that excellence has a structure and pattern linked to it. Once you understand this structure, what you're actually doing is capturing the source code of excellence. I've been a practitioner of NLP for close to two decades now, and I've realised that if you look closely, NLP is all around us. When the first carpenter taught his son how to make a chair, that was reproducing excellence, and that was NLP.

There's a 45-year-old banker Tanya whom I coached a while ago to improve her interpersonal skills, both at work and otherwise. In our very first conversation it became apparent that while it was extremely difficult for her to get along well with people, she was exceptional at certain other things. Tanya was awesome when it came to cooking. She was known among her extended family and her husband's circle of friends as "the grumpy woman who is an amazing cook." At least that's how she put it. On closer examination and questioning, it turned out that what actually made her a good cook were the following:

1. She read a lot of books and articles on cooking.
2. She cooked whenever she got a chance to.
3. She kept cooking a dish time and again till she got it absolutely right and people acknowledged that.
4. When a dish she cooked didn't come out right, she looked at it as feedback and learnt lessons from it so that she could get it right the next time around.
5. She was always smiling while she cooked, because she loved doing it.

Once Tanya understood that in an area of her life where she's excellent, she's been doing things in a certain way, she was able to compare it to how she did things when it came to people interaction. Tanya thought about this for a month and kept comparing the cooking side of her life to the people interaction side of her life. The turnaround in Tanya's interpersonal skills happened after that month when she started applying her code for cooking when she interacted with people.

1. So Tanya began to read books and articles about interpersonal skills.
2. She began to interact with people whenever she got an opportunity to.
3. If one style of communication or interaction with a person did not work, she tried another and then another, till she got the outcome she wanted.
4. When an interaction or conversation with someone didn't go well, she looked for feedback from that situation so that she could correct and improve herself.
5. Most importantly, she smiled a lot more when she interacted with people.

A combination of all these new patterns really changed the entire game for Tanya, who later started to be seen as more of a people person. So the secrets to excellence lie within you; it's just a matter of understanding and reproducing them.

And that was Arnold Schwarzenegger's response in the interview. He said that to become a successful actor, one of the major things he did was to look at his bodybuilding career. He spent time understanding what exactly he did to become Mr. Universe thrice and the I.F.B.B. Mr. Olympia seven times. He then applied the same principles to his acting career and that greatly contributed to making him a Hollywood star. So, as you approach wellbeing and make changes in your behaviour, keep in mind that you aren't trying to fix yourself. You are perfect just the way you are, and there are several things that you are already excellent in. You're just trying to spread that perfection and excellence to other sides of your being.

HOW YOU DO ANYTHING IS HOW YOU DO EVERYTHING

The above statement applies to almost all areas of your life. For example, how clean or how cluttered your desk is, could say a lot about how much clutter you can handle in your car, your room and maybe even in your life. Your approach to how you pack your luggage for a trip could say a lot about your approach to work, how you plan your weekends and about you as a person overall.

I recently coached a lady who was a middle-aged IT professional and was struggling in various areas of her life. She kept jumping jobs, changing houses, changing doctors, moving from one relationship to another and changing even hairstyles. After a detailed conversation, it was clear to me that what she lacked was consistency in her life in any area. After a bout of difficulties that she had faced in life, she was unable to regain the stability that she needed to live in peace. I suggested that she start working out and no matter what happened, to never skip a single day. She didn't see the connection between my suggestion and all the struggles in her life. We had a long discussion, and after going back and forth, she finally agreed to do it. So she registered for a fitness programme at a gym close to her house. The first month was a disaster, and she missed more days than she attended. After that, she developed a rhythm. She walked to the gym every single day, worked out for an hour and walked back. Even on Sundays.

The purpose in her case was not merely to build muscles, lose weight or reduce her waistline. The idea was to get her mind and body used to regularity. This one activity kept her anchored. She realised that she could stick with one thing and benefit from it instead of fleeing. This phenomenon of doing something regularly and consistently gradually spread to all dimensions of her life. She was in better spirits through the day and therefore started to enjoy her job more and so didn't quit when faced with the slightest concern. Her overall health and feeling of wellbeing improved due to the regular exercise and so she stopped running from one doctor to another. Her body started to become more toned, and she started to look and feel better, so didn't have the real need for a relationship or a new hairstyle to feel complete. Of course, when she started experiencing all these positive changes in her life, she began to enjoy the gym, the workouts and the new friends she made there. She didn't even want to shift houses anymore. In this lady's case, I think luck also had something to do with the results she got. But the point is that the luck never showed up till she started working out regularly.

Your dedication and commitment to one area of your life could actually be helping you learn and develop the art of being dedicated and committed in other areas of your life as well. If you want to develop a greater sense of focus in life, be more focused about one of your hobbies. If you want to learn to set and achieve big goals, set greater fitness goals for yourself and practice achieving them. You get the point.

A couple of years ago at the University of Texas, Austin, Naval Admiral William H. McRaven[22], the ninth commander of the U.S. Special Operations Command, gave a memorable speech[23]. In it he states:

"Every morning in basic SEAL training, my instructors, who at the time were all Vietnam veterans, would show up in my barracks room and the first thing they would inspect was your bed.

If you did it right, the corners would be square, the covers pulled tight, the pillow centred just under the headboard and the extra blanket folded neatly at the foot of the rack—rack—that's Navy talk for bed.

It was a simple task—mundane at best. But every morning, we were required to make our bed to perfection. It seemed a little ridiculous at the time, particularly in light of the fact that we were aspiring to be real warriors, tough battle hardened SEALs—but the wisdom of this simple act has been proven to me many times over.

If you make your bed every morning, you will have accomplished the first task of the day. It will give you a small sense of pride, and it will encourage you to do another task and another and another.

By the end of the day, that one task completed will have turned into many tasks completed. Making your bed will also reinforce the fact that the little things in life matter.

If you can't do the little things right, you will never do the big things right.

And, if by chance you have a miserable day, you will come home to a bed that is made—that you made—and a made bed gives you encouragement that tomorrow will be better."

YOU'RE ALWAYS PRACTISING

The word 'practice' gets some of us thinking about some sort of repeated performance or systematic exercise. Perhaps fields like music, dance, theatre, sport or martial arts prominently surface when we think about where practice is done the most. In reality, we are all practising something or the other all the time.

A lot of the work that I do is about understanding and using human behaviour. As I mentioned earlier, "A behaviour is anything that you do." That's one of the best definitions of behaviour that I've come across in recent times. Now all of us are practising some behaviour or the other all the time. The question is, what behaviour are you practising?

Another fact is that we get better at what we practice. If you miss your morning walk once, it is easier to miss it again. If you wake up early once, it is easier to wake up early again. There are fewer instances of people starting or stopping a behaviour in one shot. Like smoking your very first cigarette and from then on, becoming a daily smoker for the rest of your life. Or dropping out of a language class. Very few people miss one day and stop altogether. There is mostly a transition from very regular to missing a class once in a while to missing classes often to stopping altogether.

Living the good life involves regularly doing the things that will get you there. Practising the desirable behaviours more often than the undesirable ones. If you want to become a guitarist one year from now, you should be practising playing the guitar often enough for the next one year. You can't spend all your time sleeping, working, commuting, watching TV, eating or meeting friends and expect to become a guitarist after a year. I know that seems rather obvious, but that's exactly what some people do.

I recently coached a gentleman in his late thirties, who was a manager at a fairly large technology firm. He would wake up in the morning, feeling lousy about the day ahead. So he would snooze some more and wake up, not having enough time for a relaxed morning. He would then go through the discomfort of running late for office and thinking about the possible traffic jam and consequences of reaching office late. While driving to work, he would think about the long, arduous day ahead and already start feeling heavy inside. While at work, he would go about the day feeling sick about his job and wondering what he's really doing in that company. He said that when he leaves office, there's a brief period when he feels good. That is soon shrouded by thoughts of the treacherous drive back home, and when he gets home, he feels stuck with household chores and responsibilities, till he finally hits the sack. So here's someone who spends most of his day practising feeling bad.

I must admit that it might not be easy for someone like this to do a complete turnaround and start feeling elated for most of the day. In fact, what eventually worked well for him was starting with one hour a day of doing something that he loves to do, enjoying it and feeling good about it. He loved reading poetry. So he spent an hour every night reading poetry. Just taking time out for this one activity got him to look forward to getting back home after work and rush through his evening chores. After a month of doing this, I suggested that he add one more activity that he loved and that was listening to music. He started by listening to fifteen minutes of music in the morning, which he described to me as being really weird and unusual for him. He was only used to listening to music in the car or at home in the evening on TV. This was just music on his turntable. This slowly moved to thirty minutes, forty-five and then an hour. I think one of the big reasons why people hit the snooze button is because they don't look forward to the day ahead. The habit of hitting the snooze button in the morning slowly stopped for this gentleman and listening to music in the morning with his tea and the newspaper became a ritual. This was slowly spread to longer periods, coupled with redefining his life and career goals, making a job change and consciously practising feeling good every day.

The point is that people don't feel miserable overnight. It's the outcome of a lot of practice. So are feelings of wellbeing, elation and fulfilment. Go after what you want in life and practice the behaviours that will get you there.

FIVE STEPS TO A NEW BEHAVIOUR

If you've read so far, then you know that if you do something physically, like sit, stand, run, turn your head, etc., those are behaviours. If you do something in your mind, like talk to yourself, think good thoughts, make a mental plan, replay an incident, etc., those are behaviours too. Though it might not be obvious to many of us, the truth is that human beings spend most of their lives either developing new behaviours, keeping existing behaviours or getting rid of old ones. Interestingly enough, getting rid of an old behaviour, keeping an existing behaviour and developing a new behaviour are all behaviours in themselves and ones that could be developed. So the development of new behaviours becomes a significant part of living the good life. The more easily you are able to develop the kinds of behaviours that you want, the more likely you are of living your ideal life. Successful individuals from various fields like doctors, musicians, mathematicians, businessmen, martial artists and athletes know the secret to developing new behaviours extremely well. The secret is rather elementary and has five simple steps.

The first step to developing a new behaviour is to **identify exactly what the new behaviour you want to develop** is. Be clear about exactly what you will be doing if were demonstrating the new behaviour. If the new behaviour you want to develop is to start playing the guitar, nail down everything that you need to be doing to achieve that. Like the type of guitar you want to play, holding it the right way, putting your fingers on the right strings on the fretboard, strumming the guitar, the exact tune you're playing, etc. If the new behaviour you want to develop is to start walking regularly, be crystal clear about everything that you need to be doing to achieve that. Like waking up early in the morning, being clear about the exact time, getting ready and putting on your walking gear, actually stepping out of the house and beginning to walk, the exact path that you will take, what time you will finish and get back home.

The second step is to close your eyes and **see yourself doing all the things that you need to do to be demonstrating the new behaviour**. While the first step was happening at a very logical level, this step is happening at an emotional and feeling level. It, therefore, has to be done in a very calm and relaxed manner and ensuring that you experience the feelings and emotions behind all the things that you need to do. So close your eyes, consciously relax all parts of your body and slowly, when you feel your mind relaxing, see yourself going through every single detail of the new behaviour. If you're seeing yourself walking on the street, see the flowers on the trees, feel the chill air hit your face, and experience the entire walk in as much detail as possible. Do likewise for any new behaviour you want to develop.

Step three is the **practice**. You need to practice the new behaviour over and over again to get it into your system. Going for a walk for two days or being able to float on water does not make it a new behaviour. It only means that you are going in the right direction and it's not time to celebrate yet. Repeating a behaviour consciously and deliberately, over and over again, takes you to step four.

Step four is where **positive feelings about the new behaviour start to surface and eventually flood your mind.** You begin to feel good about your morning walks. You feel like walking every morning and enjoy doing it, and it's not a chore anymore. You feel confident about not just floating in the pool but moving swiftly from one end of the pool to the other. You are no more threatened by the deep end.

Step five is the final step. Here, your emotional comfort with the new behaviour becomes so high as a result of repeated practice that **the behaviour becomes rather automatic.** This realistically is the celebration time but most people who have made this journey successfully realise that reaching step five in itself is a celebration and it hardly calls for any external reward system to sustain it. But if you want to get to the top of the highest building in your city and scream in joy, totally go for it.

A GLIMPSE INTO PSYCHOLOGICAL WELLBEING

A SNAPSHOT

Wellbeing is, to a large extent, a mental game. You could be in the peak of physical health, but that just won't be called wellbeing if you're feeling depressed or gloomy. This chapter examines wellbeing through the mental wellness lens focusing on what I've commonly encountered with my clients. What's the role that your mind plays in your wellbeing? A big part of it is about looking at a person's underlying motives and ensuring that wellbeing is pursued for the right reasons. While most people don't skip food or water or even sleep, a lot of them don't pay enough attention to what they do to their minds. You'll also see in this chapter the mental equivalent of a fruit platter, a protein shake or a clean glass of water.

Sport is a great space to learn about the power of the mind and the role it plays in living the good life. I see a lot of people these days, even those who weren't open to walking into a mental hospital or signing up for psychotherapy, benefiting by dealing with some of the same issues through structured coaching sessions. Partly because the world is becoming more open to dealing with issues of the mind with less taboo attached to them and partly because coaching as a term and an intervention, sounds more empowering.

When someone like Rafael Nadal is getting coached, why not me? Some of what you'll read here are the applications of sport psychology. Particularly my personal experience in using it to help individuals in corporate organisations and elsewhere overcome their challenges.

HOW YOU SEE THE WORLD DEPENDS ON WHERE YOU ARE IN LIFE

First of all, this is not a piece that's going to give you black and white answers but is going to provoke the right questions about your worldview. I was recently discussing a mental exercise with a longtime friend and coach who also works in the field of applied psychology. Try out this exercise before you continue reading.

Ensure that you have a stopwatch with you or even a wristwatch or clock that can track time to the second. Sit in a comfortable position and as the second needle of your watch passes 12, close your eyes. You could also just close your eyes and simultaneously turn the stopwatch on. Just think about what you plan to do over the next two to three days and when you feel that exactly a minute has passed, open your eyes. Make sure you aren't trying to mentally count seconds while you do this exercise. Now look at the watch and note how much time has actually passed.

Every time I've done this exercise with people, I've had one startling observation. The people who are hurrying through life and the ones who are typically more stressed are the ones who open their eyes earlier and sometimes well before a minute. The ones who are more relaxed and are taking life with ease typically overshoot a minute by fifteen to forty-five seconds and sometimes even by an entire minute or more. I've also tried this exercise with the same person on different occasions. When people are in office, trying to get a lot of things done and meet deadlines, they open their eyes a lot sooner than a minute, and while some of the same people are on vacation or just lazing around, they tend to open their eyes well after a minute. It's not as if the one-minute mark is the tipping point on any relaxation scale. The fact is that you feel rushed, feel like there isn't enough time, feel like traffic is a hindrance, and your heart is beating faster when you have too much to do and are trying to meet strict targets. On the contrary, when you're lazing around and really have nothing in particular to get done, you feel calm, you feel like you have all the time in the world and traffic never seems to bother you.

Another classic example of people seeing the world differently depending on where they are is what happens when you're on a road trip. There might be this familiar road that you take all the time to get to your workplace or to drop your kid off at school. But when you are on a road trip with your family or a bunch of close friends, and you pass by that same familiar road, it just doesn't seem the same anymore. The feeling you get when you pass through that road is not one of monotony but of thrill and excitement instead, now that you are on a road trip. This might well start even as soon as you've driven out of your gate and into your street.

In the organisations that I've worked and consulted for in the past and even in the self-development workshops that I've conducted, I've always noticed one thing. People are in their worst moods and behaviour when they're going through shit themselves. To get a grip on this, start by being aware of the way you see the world around you because this is a great indicator of what might be going on in your body, mind and soul. Your behaviour is the user interface of your inner world with the outer. To simplify this a little more, ask yourself if you like the way your life is right now. Do you like your friends, your job, the city you live in, your situation in life, the way you spend your weekdays and weekends, your pastimes, etc.

Second, if for the most part, you like your current worldview, then you are perhaps already at peace with yourself, and that's fabulous. But if you realise that way too often or for too many days in a row, the way you see the world isn't the way you'd like it to be, then it means you probably need to change something. Third and most importantly, make those necessary changes in your life till you get to where you want to be. By that, I don't just mean change your job, your fitness level, your diet, your social circle, your city or even your wardrobe. A lot of the changes that most people need to make are within themselves, and those are the ones that ensure lasting change and will help you start seeing the world differently. In case you're wondering what those specific changes are, then you're in the right place and I'm not the one to be spelling them out to you.

WHAT MOVES YOU TO DO ANYTHING?

Have you ever wondered why we do the things that we do? What moves us? What makes us wake up in the morning and go about living our lives? Though these might seem like extremely fundamental questions, the answers are surprisingly simple. Irrespective of what your answers to the above questions are, they could fall under only two categories. There are just two broad ways in which people drive themselves in this world. In psychology, these are called intrinsic and extrinsic motivation[24].

Intrinsic motivation is the kind of motivation that comes from within. People who have a strong sense of intrinsic motivation tend to engage in activities that really interest them and experience a full sense of personal control. They constantly look into themselves for feedback on how they are doing in life. Extrinsic motivation, on the other hand, comes from an external as opposed to an internal source. Awards, praise and social approval are just some examples of such external sources. People who have a strong sense of extrinsic motivation constantly look for feedback from the outside world for whether or not they are doing well. If this idea interests you, you should go read Edward Deci and Richard Ryan's self-determination theory[25].

Because I'm more interested to talk about how this applies to almost all dimensions of life. I'd just like to highlight a few of them here.

Wealth

In the case of the creation of wealth, the extrinsically motivated individual is likely to create wealth constantly in comparison to others. It's not enough to have a big bank balance. The amount has to be considered high even by others. It's not sufficient to own a big car if everyone else has the same car and it isn't ostentatious. An intrinsically motivated person, on the other hand, is one who creates wealth for himself or herself. A certain bank balance satisfies this person purely because that is the amount that this person considers high enough to meet the purpose of having that money. An intrinsically motivated person buys a particular car or house only because that is the car or house that the person wants to own, perhaps because of the kind of technology or some internal standard.

Health

It's quite common for people who are in great health to hear some social feedback about their health and start feeling better or worse based on the feedback. This is most likely to happen to the extrinsically motivated person. An extrinsically motivated person is likely to feel bad if told that they look fat rather than an intrinsically motivated person. For an intrinsically motivated person, good health could be based more on their own personal standards of body weight, appetite, energy level, etc. Whether or not an intrinsically motivated person feels healthy is dependent on how he feels internally.

Success

What does it mean to be successful? Well, we've all heard it zillions of times that success means different things to different people. What's interesting is that for an intrinsically motivated person, success is an internal game. Which means that even after a man has great opportunities, fame, fortune and glory, he might not feel successful if his lifestyle and achievements don't match his internal model of success. An extrinsically motivated person, on the other hand, only feels successful if the people around him like his family, friends, colleagues, classmates or even enemies consider him to be a success.

The bottomline is for us to evaluate ourselves and identify where we stand on this. If you realise that you are a hugely extrinsically motivated person, then watch out to not live your life for others and end up feeling like you had a hollow victory in the end. If you realise that you are majorly an intrinsically motivated person, don't end up being unable to relate to the world around you and miss out on what others could have offered to you in life. The great danger is not that we fall into one category or the other, but that we remain there without our knowledge rather than out of choice.

WHAT DO YOU ACTUALLY WANT IN LIFE?

Why do fitness programmes have so many dropouts? Why are so many people stuck in jobs that they hate? What makes some people have unshakeable conviction about certain goals or targets that get replaced over time or vanish altogether? Think about it. The chances are that way down inside, you don't actually enjoy what you're doing. Maybe the goals that you are pursuing are not actually your goals but what you're doing for other people.

Sitting at a Robin Sharma conference a couple of years ago, I heard him say "… Join the 5 o' clock club. Wake up early; it's one of the best investments that you can make for yourself…" I realised what this man was saying was a great idea and what my parents and, for that matter, many of our parents have been telling us all along. To wake up early. I thought about this for a bit and figured that Robin Sharma made it sound far more compelling than some of our parents ever did by actually emphasising how an extra hour every day means thirty extra hours a month and that translates to 360 extra hours a year. Now if your typical workday comprises even of ten to twelve hours, then that translates to about thirty extra days a year.

But apart from all this, the reason why many people actually followed this advice is because it was Robin Sharma who was saying it. This is the age-old message-and-messenger argument that's been around forever. A lot of times, the messenger is as, if not more important than the message itself. We end up following things just because someone we respect or someone who has a powerful aura is telling us to. This sort of motivation is a good launch pad to get you to start waking up early, but it might not stop you from pressing the snooze button when the alarm goes off on the third or fourth morning.

We might land up at a concert and be so mesmerised by a band's performance that we decide to learn to play a musical instrument or take singing lessons after that. This initial wave of inspiration that gets people started is a good thing. Unfortunately, it doesn't keep many of them going for too long. Don't be trapped by the halo effect of people and practices. The fate of initiatives that you take up as a result of momentary excitement is short-lived. Habits that eventually stick and behaviours that actually develop are ones that resonate strongly with your actual desires.

At a moment when you are not struck by any kind of external motivation or inspired by any charismatic external agent, ask yourself some of these questions.

- ❖ Do I actually want to wake up early?
- ❖ Do I actually want to learn a musical instrument?
- ❖ What are the things that I actually want to do in life?

The answers that come out of such introspection are likely to be a more accurate assessment of what you really want to achieve and the things you actually want to do in life. Many of my coaching clients whom I've taken through similar exercises have ended up with a lot of clarity in terms of what they want to do and what suits them best. If walking alone every evening is a better fitness formula for you and it saves you the social discomfort of being in a gym with many people, then that's what you should do. If you've been working a job for years because your family and friends considered it to be a prestigious job, but what you actually want to do is teach, then that's what you should be doing.

What will eventually work for you is just what you actually want. There's nothing more to it.

WELLBEING DOESN'T HAVE TO BE A GAME OF CONTROL

Ask five of your closest friends or relatives what wellbeing means to them. Make a note of what they tell you. I've done this exercise myself and have heard all kinds of responses like, wellbeing is about living a happy life, wellbeing means being fit, wellbeing means not falling ill, wellbeing is being physically and mentally strong, etc. It doesn't matter what the response is. I've noticed that there is a projection of what people say into the future. Nobody wants to be happy just for the next five minutes or be mentally and physically strong just for today.

There is a definite undertone of wanting any of this along with a certain level of permanence. At the heart of the feeling of wellbeing is a need for certainty. People really want to have control over their health, their relationships, their lifespans and sometimes even the lifespans of others. A lack of control sometimes sends the lives of people spiralling downward. Just not being certain that you might have your job a month from now or that you might enjoy a healthy life for the rest of this year could cause a lot of stress and people even lose sleep over such apprehensions which, in turn, impacts their wellbeing.

People want to control all kinds of things in their lives, starting from the temperature in the room, to their weight to their blood sugar and cholesterol levels, their spouses and sometimes even the lives and futures of their children. It's no wonder that teenagers feel a sense of control and empowerment when they start working and making their own money. One of the things that any setback does is that it rattles you off your sense of control over yourself. The journey to find and experience a cure is really a journey to regain control over your life. The best diets in the world are the ones that give you the most predictable outcomes. Exercises where you can predict the number of calories lost which eventually translates into getting into the desired shape are invariably the more popular exercises. There are several parts of the world that believe in some sorts of horoscopes, oracles and prophecies, and the unsaid message from people who believe in them is, "We want to try and control our future." The whole "happily ever after" phenomenon hugely leans on the idea of taking control to reach that result.

Having control might make us all feel a little safer and secure, but it certainly isn't something to fret and fume over. Sometimes it's good to let go because the fact is that stock markets do fluctuate, economies do collapse, and people eventually do fall sick or die. Don't be so obsessed with trying to gain control of life that it starts controlling you. Your relationship with life is like any other relationship. The more controlling you get, sometimes the less control you actually end up having. To quote the Chicago Tribune columnist Mary Schmich[26] once more,

"Don't worry about the future. Or worry, but know that worrying is as effective as trying to solve an algebra equation by chewing bubble gum. The real troubles in your life are apt to be things that never crossed your worried mind, the kind that blindside you at 4 p.m. on some idle Tuesday."

WHAT YOU SEE IS EXACTLY WHAT YOU GET

I'd like to quote Arnold Schwarzenegger one more time, "Bodybuilding is much like any other sport. To be successful, you must dedicate yourself 100% to your training, diet and mental approach." For any dimension of wellbeing, one such mental approach worth dedicating yourself to is visualisation.

When you embark on a fitness journey to go from where you are to where you want to be, the following two steps are rudimentary.

The first step is to know exactly where you are right now in terms of fitness. This is your current reality. It can be done by fairly sophisticated methods like DEXA (Dual Energy X-ray Absorptiometry), BODPOD, BodyMerix, Bio Electrical Impedance, etc. to measure body composition and body fat. Alternately, simply use the more old school but still working methods like callipers, measuring tapes, weighing scales or even just looking at yourself in the mirror. You could also consider getting "Before" pictures of yourself taken.

The second and more important step is to visualise how you would look when you reach your ideal fitness level. What do you see when you look into the mirror or when you get your photographs taken? Making a mental image of your ideal or desired self is an extremely powerful part of you being able to achieve your fitness goals. This approach applies as well to weight loss as it does to weight gain or to gaining strength or even in enhancing performance as an athlete of any kind.

You could use this in any area of your life by spending ten minutes practising this routine.

1. Close your eyes and relax your entire body. During this time breathe normally and deliberately and consciously relax all the muscles of your body from head to toe.

2. Now make an image of yourself in your ideal state. Having already achieved what you want to achieve. Let this image be as clear and explicit as possible. Visualise every detail and see all the related tangible and intangible resources around you in your ideal state.

3. As you visualise, engage with your mental image using all your senses. If you're imagining a fancy dinner for a group of friends in your new mansion. See it clearly in your mind's eye, see the faces of the people around the table, hear the sounds as you walk in through the different rooms, hear the conversations and the voices of your guests, smell the aroma of the food in the air, taste the different dishes and relish them, and feel the world around you, the chair you're sitting on, the ground beneath your feet, the cutlery you're holding and the hugs and kisses of the people who've come home.

4. Once you've done this long enough and if you've done it right, you'd be feeling a sense of delight inside you. Now bring your awareness back to the present moment and slowly open your eyes.

5. You might open your eyes and tell yourself, "Well, I still don't own that mansion nor have those friends over for that fancy dinner." That's alright. Remember that visualisation is not the same as teleportation. Once you open your eyes and if you've done the routine right, you'll feel warm and fuzzy inside. You will have a sense of knowing that you don't have it yet but it's coming.

The advantage of following this visualisation routine every day is twofold. It gives your mind a clear goal to work towards. As a result, each time you do an activity, your mind subconsciously knows where it is headed. It also awakens the R.A.S. or Reticular Activation System[27], a part of the brain that is responsible for regulating arousal and sleep-wake transitions. In this case what the R.A.S. does is that it helps you identify the resources that are required to reach your ideal life. These could be your ideal fitness trainer, the right job opportunity, a new business idea or even just an unexplained drive to work harder and with more zest for anything you take up. Whatever ensures that you live into the mental movie that you watched.

WATCHING YOUR MENTAL NUTRITION

Most people start pursuing any goal in life because they were inspired by something they saw, read, heard about or even imagined. This is a phenomenon similar to people walking out of a theatre after watching Sherlock Holmes and feeling like detectives themselves. Unfortunately, inspiration is also the trigger for many a short-lived endeavour.

The world of sport is filled with examples of athletes who grew rapidly in their sport at the start but could not reach the top or could not stay on top for long once they got there. This applies to all areas of life. What got you into a pursuit won't necessarily keep you there. In other words, you might have started pursuing a certain goal as a result of a specific kind of inspiration of a certain intensity. You might have been inspired to start working out after meeting an old classmate whose body is still in such good shape while you had let yourself slack and gain weight. You might have registered for a martial arts programme after watching a demonstration by experts from the Shaolin temple and being inspired by the grace and agility of the human body. You could have drawn inspiration from an older relative who ran a full marathon at the age of 75, and then taken up running yourself. This starting dose of inspiration does just that. It just gets you started. It's mostly not sufficient to keep you going because as you move along and days pass, this initial shot of inspiration will fade away.

Like you fuel your body with the right food, water, vitamins and roughage, it's critical to fuel the mind with its required dose of inspiration. What nutrition is to the body, inspiration is to the mind. Just like you wouldn't skip a meal or allow your body to dehydrate due to a lack of water intake, don't let your mind get bored and demotivated due to a lack of inspiration. You'll be amazed by what inspiration can make people do. Nourish your mind with inspiration by trying out any or all of the following. I've used fitness, an area where the dropout rates are among the highest, as one example. The other example is related to different professions, an area of life where a lot of people are trying to get better.

- ❖ Read books or watch videos about your fitness area especially seeking to learn more. Expertise creates interest. If you want to start a restaurant in your city, read and watch videos about the best restaurants in the world and how they got started.
- ❖ Keep your eyes open for success stories of people in your fitness area. If they can do it, you can do it. If you want to start your own business, read about the success stories of people who've done that from scratch. Perhaps even read about the ones who did it with limited or no initial investment.
- ❖ Join groups and fora or attend seminars and conferences related to your fitness area. A lot of people do something just because that's what

they stand for. If you want to become a better investor, attend conferences or seminars related to investment or even attend workshops conducted by the investment gurus.

❖ Speak to role models in your fitness area and find out what drives them. There are a precious few drivers that inspire most of us. If you're trying to become a CEO, reach out to people who are already CEOs, try to schedule a meeting with them or take them out for breakfast and ask them what you need to know. Ask them to mentor you.

❖ Follow the lives and careers of the best people in your area of fitness. The best people in any field are charismatic and inspire others toward action. If you want to become a good photographer, look at what the best photographers out there are doing. Watch documentaries on them or watch their interviews. Explore what they're working on right now and what they think is the next big idea.

Remember, there are very few instances in the world of people quitting before their inspiration runs dry.

DEVELOPING MENTAL TOUGHNESS

As I was working on a psychology research project on how I would personally define mental toughness, I thought about some of the people who I think are mentally tough. Andre Agassi, Lance Armstrong, Oprah Winfrey, Steve Jobs, Nick Vujicic, Vincent Van Gogh, Will Smith in the movie *Pursuit of Happiness* (which is based on Chris Gardner's life), Admiral William McRaven, Ruth Beitia and a few other people I know personally, either through work or otherwise. My definition is based on qualities that they possess.

Mental toughness is the ability of a person to achieve what he or she sets out to achieve despite opposition or hardships and ensure that setbacks, unexpected circumstances, lack of ability, lack of support from others, physical and mental discomfort, uncertainty and defeat are dealt with and overcome systematically. This is done by taking specific steps, getting better and moving closer to the ultimate goal while enjoying the process of doing it.

Here are a few ways in which I've helped people develop mental toughness. If you want to develop mental toughness, this is what you should do.

1. Never simplify your goals or dreams for the future for fear that you might not achieve them or because at some point it seems like too much hard work, too much pain, it looks overwhelming or for any other such reason.

2. Always wake up before or exactly at the time that you decided the previous night. Never later.

3. Make your bed perfectly as soon as you wake up, even before you go to the toilet, brush your teeth or drink water. If required, dust the bedspread, fold the blanket or stretch out the pillow cover. But ensure that your bed is in perfectly set condition and ready for you to sleep before you leave its side in the morning.

4. Meditate for at least thirty minutes following any specific meditation practice that suits your taste. Ideally, pick a meditation practice that requires you to sit in one position and meditate.

5. Make a list of the top five things that you need to achieve before the end of each day, which will make that day a successful and fruitful day for you. Review this to-do list once every hour till the workday ends.

6. Do anything only because you want to do it. Never succumb to any kind of compulsion. Never do anything because the feeling of wanting to do it is so strong and almost uncontrollable. This could be related to wanting to eat chocolate, smoking a cigarette, watching TV, calling someone on the phone, etc.

7.   Make a list of the things that you love to eat or drink and give up one thing from that list for a month. Do this for a different item each month.

8.   Three times a week, when you feel like acting impulsively on something, just wait for an hour before you actually act. The purpose of this is to strengthen your mind and not to torture your body. So don't do things like not drinking water for an hour when you are really tired and feeling dehydrated. Use this on things like wanting to call someone to find out what happened with their interview or wanting to open the parcel from Amazon to see the new book you ordered.

9.   One morning a week, reflect on the week that went by and identify any pending decision on any issue from the previous week. Make a decision to follow a specific course of action on that issue and follow through with it in the week that follows. Don't push it beyond that.

10.   Workout for at least thirty minutes a day, either in the morning or in the evening. Do a combination of freehand or weight-training exercises that you find useful.

11.   At the end of each day before you go to bed, write down three wins or three victories that you had on that day. It doesn't matter how small those wins are.

12.   Don't ever stop doing something that is taking you closer to your goal just because it is uncomfortable or difficult to do. Keep at it.

13. Only pursue goals that you really want to achieve and ones that make sense to you. Don't pursue a goal for anyone else or one that doesn't make sense to you.

14. Lastly, don't try to follow each and every one of the above tips to the T. Pick any seven that make sense to you but stick with them.

As you follow the above points and become mentally tougher, remember that mental toughness is not what you exercise when things are going smooth, and you are getting what you want in life. The time when things are going smooth might be a good time to develop mental toughness, but that's unlikely to be when you use it. Your mental toughness is like a sustained release drug. It does its job mostly when the pain or symptom shows itself up. It is the quality that you carry that helps you get through turbulent times due to any of the reasons mentioned in my earlier definition. Mental toughness is what defines you when things are not going your way.

A PLACE WHERE NO ONE AND NOTHING CAN AFFECT YOU

In case you haven't heard the story of the Zen master and the earthquake[28], here it is. A Zen master was having dinner one evening with his disciples. A major earthquake struck, and while everything shook and swayed, the disciples ran frantically to other rooms and to different parts of the monastery. Some even ran right out of the monastery in an attempt to save their lives. In a while, the earthquake settled down and the tremors stopped. So the disciples started to find their way back to the monastery and eventually into the room where the dinner was served. They found the Zen master still seated in silence with a calm and peaceful look on his face. When the disciples asked him how come he didn't run out to save his life, he replied that the quake was everywhere. In that room, the next room and even outside the monastery. So the only place you could actually escape to was into yourself. That's what the Zen master did.

We sometimes don't realise that we all have access to a place like this. A room where no one and nothing can affect you. A place where you can be in a state of absolute bliss despite the earthquakes and hurricanes of life that might surround you. But before you start gaining access to this room you need to identify it and if you can't do that, at least build one for yourself.

There are some of us who are lucky enough to have found that sacred space early on in life. Either by practising a form of art or music or meditation or through writing or even just by knowing how to relax in our own way. These are the people who almost have a readymade room, and the journey they take is just about drifting gracefully in their mental or spiritual space into that room. Let's also accept the fact that some of us might have come into this world without a blessed space to go to or might be so far removed from that peaceful room that it's far smarter for us to build a new one from scratch. Here's what you should do if you want to build your own room of bliss.

Spend time every day doing something that you absolutely love. Read a book, workout, take a walk in the park, write, practice martial arts, go on a bike ride, meditate or do whatever else that makes you feel good. Try to pick activities that take you inward rather than keep you distracted from your inner self and take you further away from your centre. So things like drinking, drugs, gambling, gaming or television could be bad options. When you do the things you love often enough, you'll notice that the intensity of the good feeling that you experience starts to expand and become more powerful. That's when you realise that your room is slowly getting built.

You'll notice that some activities work better for you than others. For some, meditating for an hour might get them into a quiet and serene space while for some others, sitting in a café reading a book for a while might make them feel tranquil. Choose what works best for you and stick with it. This is like finding the right entrance to your serene space. Repeat your favourite activity frequently. This does not mean quitting your job and doing it all the time. There is great power in spaced repetition. Each time you enter your peaceful room, the more definite it becomes. First, you identify a spot, then you mark it, then the walls get built, then the ceiling and interiors and lights and fragrances. The more often you go into this room, the more robust your room becomes.

A final thought is that once you identify your room or build one for yourself, don't abandon it. I've met a lot of people who've had a really calm mental space that they could go to whenever they wanted to. One that their parents inculcated or ushered them into or perhaps one that they themselves identified in the process of growing up. But as they grew older and got caught up in the natural disasters of everyday life, they stopped going to this room and eventually this room got abandoned or forgotten altogether. Finally, at some point when they have a midlife crisis or experience severe job stress, they don't know where to go.

So once you know your safe haven, respect it, guard it and enjoy it for life. It's a place where nothing can affect you.

WHAT ARE YOU CONSTANTLY TELLING YOURSELF

A SNAPSHOT

Irrespective of which culture you belong to, the power of stories is indispensable. A lot of these stories are what you hear while growing up, from your parents or grandparents or other people around you. This eventually gets replaced by what you hear in the news or read in the newspaper. There are brands and organisations and cities and entire cultures that are trying to tell their stories and, obviously, as an individual, you have your own story too. Not only do you have your own story, but you also keep telling yourself different things based on your story. People around you can never be part of your life without being subject to some parts of your story. Most importantly, you are subjecting your life to your own story in deep and powerful ways. The dialogue to your story is the constant voiceover to the thoughts that cross your mind. The Zen Buddhists refer to this as the Monkey Mind or the Mental Chatter[29].

This chapter is essentially about the relationship between this chatter, wellbeing and who you are as a person. While I'm at it, I've also examined a lot of the chatter that surrounds people and impacts their wellbeing, which comes from external influences. What you keep telling yourself and the underlying story is a good reflection of who you are, and changing this story is a great way to move into the life of your dreams or into greater wellbeing.

YOU CAN SHUT UP, BUT YOU JUST CAN'T STOP COMMUNICATING

Communication is the manner in which our stories show themselves up in our lives. Since we are subject to our own stories and the stories of others, understanding a few of the nuances of communication is a great starting point to building better stories. A lot of literature on communication talks about how human communication starts from the moment a child is born and goes on till a person's last breath. The truth is that the actual process of communication starts well before the child is born, almost from the moment of conception. The embryo communicates its presence to the mother through chemical changes in the body with related mood and emotional implications. The growing mass of cells communicates the need for a certain kind of care for the mother. The unborn baby, on the verge of entering the big wide world, communicates through the mother, by sending her into labour.

Communication, being such a fundamental element of human existence, continues to play a crucial role throughout a person's life. While the difference between verbal and non-verbal communication is common knowledge for most people, it's still not uncommon for people who want to stop communicating with someone else to merely stop talking to them. In fact, silence is one of the most powerful modes of communication. A few seconds of silence in a conversation or a dramatic pause can sometimes convey far more than several minutes of dialogue. Not only can silence convey a person's unwillingness to communicate but it can also convey a person's real emotions. Feelings of anger, shame, guilt, bliss, comfort and discomfort can be conveyed through silence.

Another close cousin of silence in the arena of communication is absence. People who don't turn up for a meeting, an interview or even to office on a particular day convey a lot through their absence. Even going late for any work appointment communicates a lot about your punctuality and sometimes your work ethics, to the person who you've kept waiting. Party hosts in social occasions remember the guests who didn't show up for the party, long after the occasion is over. Friends, colleagues and family members sometimes spend hours discussing others who aren't even there to share the moment. Many a times, your absence speaks much louder than your presence.

There are also the quiet ones who think their communication is best demonstrated through their actions. What they do, the way they care for others, the commitments they live up to and the overall behaviour they demonstrate. While there's no debate on the fact that your actions are a powerful mode of communication, the point that is often missed out is the communicating power of inaction. Restaurants that are given poor feedback by their customers and don't do anything about it communicate their "We Don't Care" attitude. People who get blamed for no fault of theirs but don't speak up or clarify their point, communicate their low level of self-respect. People who have dreams and aspirations but don't take any action towards realising them communicate their laziness or poor appetite for life.

Another factoid is that the process of communication doesn't stop with your last breath. Dead people communicate the need to be put to rest by others. Their absence, in turn, communicates the need for their loved ones to make adjustments and move on. Obituary messages and posthumous awards and recognitions are other classic examples of how your communication could outlive you.

The point I'd like to make is that this is the nature of communication. It's non-stop. Likewise, what you keep telling yourself in your head or what I referred to as Mental Chatter earlier is also how you communicate to yourself. It's a non-stop process. The idea is not to stop it but to channelise it sensibly, and in any case, stopping the chatter won't ensure that the communication stops.

WHAT'S YOUR WELLBEING STORY?

We create our own stories about who we are and believe in them like they are the gospel truth. Meaning, we live into our own stories. If you want to enhance your wellbeing, create stories that support good health and wellness.

Most of us are already aware that for good health and wellbeing one needs regular exercise, a healthy diet, lots of water, a job that you enjoy, relationships that you relish and enough rest, to name a few. But several stories that we create about ourselves actually end up working against our wellbeing. These stories could be mere labels that we give ourselves or ideas that we believe in and repeat to ourselves and others. For example: I'm A Foodie, I'm A Beer Guzzler, I'm A Chain Smoker, I Drink Like A Fish, I'm A Couch Potato, I'm A Workaholic, etc.

A person who brands himself as a "foodie" actually starts to live into that story and is more likely to be the one who eats the most in his group. A person who calls himself a "beer guzzler" or claims to "drink like a fish" might perhaps find a compelling need to be the last one to be holding his drink at any party.

Developing beliefs and stories that support wellbeing can be done by following what I call the "Realise and Replace" method.

The starting point to any behaviour change is to have the self-awareness and **realise** the different unhealthy stories that you might have created for yourself. For any unhealthy habit that you have, look for the story that might be driving it. For instance, the habit of smoking a few cigarettes every day could have different stories behind it. For instance, smoking helps me relax, all managers in my organisation smoke, smoking helps me think better, my grandfather smoked till he was 93, etc. These stories mostly have different feelings or emotions that they trigger, like happiness, pride, uniqueness, belongingness, security, etc.

The second step is to **replace** this with a new story that could help you trigger the same feeling or emotion and practice the related healthy behaviour. For example: Running or even a brisk walk helps me relax, I am the only manager here who is bold enough to not smoke, a glass of chilled water calms me down and helps me think better, I could quit smoking now and live a healthier and longer life than my grandfather, etc.

In essence, spot your unhealthy and self-destructive stories and abandon them completely. Create new labels, new ideas and in turn new stories for yourself and live into them. Rest assured that you stand a much higher chance of getting fitter by replacing "I'm a foodie" with "I'm a fitness enthusiast," replacing "I'm always the last man drinking at any party" with "I have fun at parties and leave when I feel like," replacing "I'm a couch potato" or "I'm a workaholic" with "I'm a martial artist" or "I lead a balanced life."

One of my clients, Vivek, once asked me, "Is it that simple? That I just have to identify my lousy story and find a new and awesome story for myself?" Well here's exactly what I got him to do. His story was "smoking is cool." I asked him to make a note of how many times this story surfaces in his head each day. That's the first thing to do. Just notice the number of times that story surfaces. In his case, it was between fifteen and twenty times. The next thing we did together was to get a new and more empowering new story. This story was called "I am cool." It was the outcome of a lot of discussion on his qualities, what makes him unique, his ability to speak well, his competencies at work, his network of friends, etc.

Even the Alcoholics Anonymous[30], one of the most well-known and successful habit-changing organisations in the world, works because it forces people to identify the cues and the rewards that encourage their alcoholic habits and then helps them find new behaviours. For him, smoking was a way to feel cool among his colleagues, his friends and new acquaintances. So he started with once every day. When he was about to dance to the tune of the "Smoking is Cool" story, he exercised one of his other qualities that made him cool. So when he was at a bar with friends, instead of lighting a cigarette, he started sharing an interesting incident from his life that happened the previous week. Everyone laughed, and he felt good. This was the "I am cool" story at play. When he was on a coffee break with a colleague, instead of smoking, he shares with his colleague, a solution for a problem that the colleague is facing at work. The colleague is awed by the way Vivek thinks and thanks him for the solution. This makes him feel important. Another expression of the "I am cool" story. Vivek kept replacing each instance of the "smoking is cool" story with the "I am cool" story, and this changed a lot of things for him. He greatly reduced the number of cigarettes he smokes. He particularly remembers smoking a lot when he was waiting for someone. Being made to wait made him feel very uncool and smoking was his antidote to it. He still smokes a cigarette once in a while, but now it's not to make himself feel any cooler. It's just to enjoy the flavour of the cigarette with his drink.

YOU BECOME WHAT YOU TALK ABOUT

Try this simple experiment. Record the things you say for an entire day, starting from when you wake up in the morning until you go to bed at night. You could use a Dictaphone, your mobile phone or any other recording device to do this. Once you're done, review the recording and make a note of the kind of words that you've used as well as the different themes that you've discussed through the day. Consider doing this for a week, and you might surprise yourself with the things you find out about what you talk about. People I've suggested this to in the past have made a remarkable difference in their levels of wellbeing and in their lives overall. Here's what I've observed.

The kind of words you use has a serious impact on your wellbeing. You can attract certain ailments as well as life situations based on what you talk about and the words you use to talk about them. People often use phrases like

- ❖ I can't handle this
- ❖ Gosh! Not again
- ❖ I'm stressed
- ❖ I'm under a lot of pressure
- ❖ I'll never get this right

❖ I can't complete this
❖ I'm losing it
❖ I can't take this anymore
❖ Now I'm screwed
❖ I'm useless

The power of the words you use is so huge that repeating phrases like the ones above actually has a negative impact on your level of confidence and eventually your performance. Richard Cox, in his book on the concepts and applications of Sport Psychology[31], talks about the importance of positive self-talk and how specific affirmation statements can lead to higher levels of confidence and, in turn, performance. In it, he specifically states what different athletes could use. A goalie in soccer could say, "Nothing gets by me." A server in tennis might use, "I can hit a strong and accurate first serve." A golfer could repeat, "I have the perfect swing." I'm sure you get the picture. I've observed among the people I've coached in the corporate world that repeating self-defeating statements to themselves drops their confidence in what they're trying to get done and that, in turn, impacts the way they do them.

Another thing to watch out for when you listen to your recording is the kind of information that you're reporting or discussing in your conversations. Try asking five different people you know about what's happening in their lives. You'll notice that some people spontaneously start discussing their poor health, their unfortunate life situation, the increasing pollution, poverty and every other thing that's going wrong in the world. Guess what? They become what they talk about. These are the people who attract more of these negative situations into their lives so that they can talk about them and also attract the people who want to partake in these discussions. Low levels of wellbeing and negativity are likely to be recurrent themes in the lives of such people. On the contrary, there are some people who spontaneously start talking about things that are exciting, upbeat and wonderful in their lives. These people invariably attract the good life, success and happiness into their lives along with the people they could discuss them with. In either case, you get more of what you talk about. And I must add, talk about sincerely. If you talk about good health and prosperity, but you actually don't believe in it, you attract nothing.

Try this, and you are bound to attract the good life. Examine the words that you use and eliminate completely the words that imply a lack of ability, motivation, competence or confidence. Better still, replace these words with words that are more positive and empowering. Instead of saying "I'm losing it" or "Gosh! Not again," you could say something like "I've got this under control" or "Alright! I've done this before."

Spot the recurrent themes that you keep discussing and the people you keep discussing them with. I understand it could be difficult to eliminate the negative people from your life, but what you can certainly do is eliminate the negative themes. The next time someone asks you about what's happening in your life, make a focused effort of identifying, reporting and discussing what's going well in your life, as there's always something going well. The more you talk about it, the more it spreads to all other areas of your life.

LITERAL LISTENING – KNOW WHAT'S REALLY RUNNING THROUGH YOUR HEAD

Many books on communication talk about the importance of listening and techniques to listen more effectively. Some common techniques that are typically discussed include:

- ❖ Face the person
- ❖ Make eye contact
- ❖ Respond verbally
- ❖ Respond non-verbally
- ❖ Paraphrase
- ❖ Ask questions
- ❖ Don't try to provide solutions, etc.

While all this is quite useful to help someone listen better, the real solutions to a person's problems come by moving to the next level of listening. This is what I call Literal Listening. Literal Listening is about listening exactly to the choice of words that people use when they speak to you and taking them at face value.

I was recently coaching a senior corporate executive to overcome some of his work-related challenges and be more effective while in office. One of his big challenges was that he couldn't get to the most critical areas of work or the most crucial tasks that would give him maximum results in the shortest time. So in my coaching conversation with him, these are exactly some things he said and how he said them to me:

- ❖ "I come into office. One thing happens after another and by the time I deal with them, the day gets over."
- ❖ "When I try to do what I most need to do, nothing seems to be in place."
- ❖ "I never end up doing the most critical tasks."
- ❖ "I see new assignments and deadlines coming towards me in an uncontrollable manner."

Statements like the above made a few things crystal clear about his beliefs, mindset and feeling about work.

- ❖ Firstly, he feels that what is happening at the office is completely out of his control.
- ❖ Secondly, he does not pilot himself through the activities of the day but sort of floats around from one task to another.
- ❖ Thirdly, he sees the most critical tasks as ones that he needs to end up doing as a result of other circumstances rather than directing himself towards those tasks out of his own will.
- ❖ Fourthly, he believes that new assignments and deadlines cannot be controlled by him.

This is a classic case of a person facing certain challenges in life that he cannot solve but tells you clearly what is happening inside his head and leaves you with useful clues to help in solving them.

What eventually helped this corporate executive was a series of coaching sessions that first of all helped him establish the fact that he is in control of his work and not the other way around. To help him internalise this idea and produce tangible results, we started with gaining control over small tasks at work and then moved on to more complex ones. The next step was to start planning and prioritising more effectively so that the most critical factors are addressed before anything else. Once again, starting with small areas of work and eventually being able to exercise prioritisation over all areas of work in his span of control.

And coming to think of it, this whole transformation was possible by literally listening to what exactly he was telling me at the start and how he was saying it, which opened doors to the actual problems underlying his challenges.

THE TRUTH ABOUT WELLBEING ADVICE

We've spoken so far about what we tell ourselves and how to listen to what might be going on in our heads. There are also a lot of things that the world around us throws at us – what I refer to as the external chatter. This external chatter sometimes becomes what we replay in our heads and talk about later to others.

Whether it's working out in a gym, ordering healthy food at a restaurant or dealing with the day-to-day challenges of life, unsolicited advice is inevitable and often comes to us from all directions. This sort of advice on anything and everything under the sun mostly comes free, since for many, even just the habit of giving unsolicited advice to others is second nature. If you happen to be on the receiving end of such advice, remember that from a wellbeing perspective, our bodies and minds are unique machines and what works for one person might not necessarily work for another.

The world is filled with contradictory theories and research findings. People believed for centuries that the earth was the centre of the universe. Though, when Nicolaus Copernicus came along in the early 16th century and proved that the sun was, in fact, the centre of the universe and not the earth, everything changed. The health industry is filled with such instances. There is interesting research that shows that a certain number of cups of coffee a day is bad for health and another research from somewhere else that shows that the same number of cups of coffee a day is good. There was a time when in many parts of Europe, olive oil was considered bad and now it is considered as one of the safer oils to use for food. Scientific research keeps proving what was considered good so far as bad and vice versa. Unfortunately, a lot of such research findings translate into advice for better wellbeing.

Another interesting source of such advice is what I call 'family/hand-me-down' advice. Members of our family tell us different things at different points of time, and this often sticks in our minds, and some of us even live by them. I've met families that believe that drinking milk at night is good and families that believe that it is absolutely bad. Here are a couple of other interesting contradictions. Hot water showers are good versus always shower in cold water. Don't eat fruits when you have a bad stomach versus shift to a fruit diet if you have a bad stomach. You can drink as much water as you like versus drinking too much water drains your body of its essential minerals and vitamins.

Follow these tips to deal with this advice phenomenon better in your own life.

- ❖ When advice comes to you, listen to it, make a mental note of it and evaluate it using your discretion.
- ❖ Don't counter-attack, especially if the advice clashes with your own idea of truth or your own personal

wellbeing philosophy. Ask questions if required to understand the advice and its credibility better.

❖ Do your research and speak to experts (though research findings could change).

❖ When you don't agree with someone else's advice, evaluate your philosophy. Maybe you're sticking to certain rules because that's what your parents told you or because that's what you've always done.

❖ Make your own decision and do what works best for your body and mind.

In the world we live in, free advice can only be managed but not eradicated altogether. Because apart from the people we interact with, there is an entire industry of websites, publications and videos that thrive on it. Pick and use what resonates with your own version of the truth and for the rest, consider the two things that Oscar Wilde said in two different pieces of his work.

"It is always a silly thing to give advice, but to give good advice is absolutely fatal."

"The only thing to do with good advice is to pass it on. It is never of any use to oneself."

HOW THE INTERNET DECIDES YOUR HEALTH AND WELLBEING

Apart from the usual part that the internet plays as the information superhighway, there are several roles that it's taken up in the 21st Century. The internet could be your counsellor, doctor, dietician, medical dictionary and sometimes even your fitness instructor or life coach. People seek answers to various dimensions of wellbeing on the internet, from ways to lose weight to how to overcome depression.

Here are a couple of typical instances.

Imagine a man in his forties who lives in one of our big cities who suddenly starts to experience a chest pain. Now many jobs in these cities are high-pressure jobs and the natural tendency for the person is to link this chest pain to a possible indication of a heart attack. So he goes online to one of the search engines and searches for "symptoms of heart attack." The internet obviously throws out various symptoms of a heart attack and one of them topping the list is a chest pain. If he had searched instead for "causes of chest pain," he would have come across a range of other possibilities like lung-related problems, gastrointestinal problems, hypertension or sometimes even muscle injury that causes chest pain. If nothing else, this at least diffuses the tension that builds up in the person who thinks he's having a heart attack.

Now imagine a techie. A woman in her late thirties who works for a leading IT firm. She starts to feel a looming numbness in one of her arms. She thinks she is having a stroke, so she goes online and searches for "symptoms of a stroke" and sure enough, she finds "numbness in the arm" to be one of them. This convinces her even more that she might actually be having a stroke. This is not taking away from the fact that people need to get medical help when they have a health problem. The point is that if you've already decided that you are having a stroke and go about searching for and doing things that support that belief, guess what? Even if you don't have a real stroke, you'll be pumping yourself with all sorts of negative information and feeling lousy about what might happen. If this woman had approached the situation more neutrally and searched instead for "reasons for numbness in the arm," she might have come across a host of other possibilities like cervical spondylitis, fracture, panic or even using the computer for extended periods and having her wrist jammed against the edge of the table while using the mouse.

If you've been eating spinach regularly and you search for "health benefits of spinach" on the internet, that's exactly what you'll find. However, if someone suddenly tells you that spinach is not too good for health and you go online and look for "dangers of eating spinach," you will sure enough find reasons to stop eating spinach altogether. Try searching online for the ten best exercises to get six-pack abs and ten exercises to avoid a bad back, and you'll see clear overlaps.

The idea is to make decisions that support good health and wellbeing rather than scan the internet for reasons that might support poor health. Many a times, people are merely looking for reasons to support a decision that they've already made in their minds. To make informed choices about your health and wellbeing, don't make decisions and then collect evidence to support it. Collect evidence, do your research and then make your decisions.

CREATE AN AWESOME STORY FOR YOUR LIFE

When people I meet through work talk to me about their lives and the problems that they face, there are a couple of things that stand out. One is their general outlook to life. There could be someone else who is facing exactly the same problems but doesn't see them as problems at all. They might see them as challenges that help them learn and grow. The second and more important thing that stands out is their story. Not just the story that they're telling me but the story that they're telling themselves and the whole world and the one they've bought into completely. Since, in either case, we all create stories and live into them, we might as well create some awesome stories for our lives. Here's how you could do that.

And by the way, write all this down. This is not just a thinking exercise, it's a writing exercise. At the same time, this is not meant to be a test of your writing skills. The key is to get your storyline and significant events in place.

Start by creating what I call a "signature" for your story. A theme. What do you really stand for? If somebody was to read your story, what would be the one big lesson from it? Some poor signatures include, "life is a struggle, and God throws them at you for a reason," "I need to be a righteous person, no matter what," "There's no such thing as happiness, just accept that and move on," etc. While in very specific contexts in life, these could make sense, in the larger scheme of things, I've noticed that the people who've told me of such signatures have resigned to a life of struggle and dissatisfaction. Some good signatures include, "Everyday is a glide through your blessings," "You can get anything you want if you do the right things," "Life gets easier and more meaningful with each passing day" and "Basking in the bliss." These are signatures that have hope, that are prepared for good times and that push people toward positive action.

Move into the next part which is about "defining the hero." You are obviously the hero of your story. This is something that you just have to accept. I've met some people who are not comfortable playing the lead role in their stories. Remember, this is not a community story. This is your story, and you are the centre of this story. In any case, it's not like this story is going to soon be screened on popular channels across the world. This is a very personal exercise, and you are likely to be the only one reading this story, unless you decide to share it with others. The "defining the hero" step is about nailing down at least five awesome qualities or resources that you have as a hero and then five more qualities or resources that you would like to have. So, ten in total. These are the virtues that you already possess or want to develop soon. These could also be anything from your sense of humour, your education, a person or people who are always by your side, the city you live in, your communication skills, your networking ability, any other ability you possess or even the fact that you are born into a certain kind of family.

A quick note on identifying qualities or resources. Most importantly, this is an exercise by and for you. A fundamental expectation when you do this is to be brutally honest with yourself. The only thing you need to report here is the truth, without worrying about what it might look like to somebody else. Because here, there is no "somebody else." Also, remember to ask yourself some elementary questions. For example, if you were a successful architect in Mumbai, you might ask yourself, "What really got me to this position?" You would probably get answers like, education, lovely parents, people know me in this city, I have great clients, I'm hardworking, etc. Then you could go one level deeper and ask yourself, "How come I landed up in this city or got this good education or have such good clients?" That's going to throw up more answers, and you could keep going this way. Then it's just a process of shortlisting the top qualities and resources you have.

The next step is to "define the villains." The important point to keep in mind here is that the villains are not people. Because even in real life, people are rarely the real villains. It's often qualities within ourselves that make it difficult to deal with certain people, who we, therefore, see as villains. If, for instance, you are easily irritable, then anyone could seem like a villain to you. So the villains could be your vices, certain scenarios, the economy, your life situation, poor decisions you've made, etc. Include up to ten villains from the current viewpoint of your life. Once you've defined the hero and the villains, move on to the next step.

This step is where your ability to connect the dots and create the story comes into the picture. Use some of Walt Disney's tips[32] to formulate your story.

* Allow good to win over evil through the hero's virtues.
* Basic morality should inform your story.
* Never manipulate or add excessive emotion without cause.
* Don't allow your storytelling to become wishy-washy or run-of-the-mill. Know what you want to express and do so in a unique way.
* Don't allow cynicism to enter your writing.
* Develop your story toward a satisfying ending. What will make it a happy ending?

As you write this out, paint a picture of the challenges that you're facing right now in life and how you effectively use your different virtues and resources or develop new abilities to overcome them. This is a big part of your story.

The last step of the process is called "Relish Life." One of the things that I hated about the movie *The Pursuit of Happiness* is that, in the movie, there's hardly any happiness. Let your story not be like that. Remember that your story doesn't have to be a series of villains showing up one after another and you as the hero winning over those situations by using your virtues. Spend time in your story on the actual happiness part. What happens when all your villains are killed, and your challenges are overcome? Do you arrive? If you don't, then make sure you arrive. Spend adequate time and space in your story to describe your ideal life where you have everything you want, and you're living, loving and relishing them. Remember to enjoy the journey towards that ideal life. This will help you to also relish where you are, for you are on the right path and the next step will only result in greater happiness. Describe in as much detail as possible what your life would look like then. Your lifestyle, the people in your life, the kind of place you live in, how you spend your time and most importantly, how all that makes you feel. At this stage, look back at your signature and see if your story fits the bill. If not, make the necessary changes in your story so that it lives up to the theme. Since this was a creation process, if your story has turned out to be so brilliant that you want to go back and change the signature, then do that. The idea is for you to love your signature, the story and how things turn out in it.

Once you've done this, print this story out and keep it at your desk or save a copy of it in your laptop or phone. Make sure you read through the entire story at least once a week. You'll be amazed at how you start to make changes in your life, make new decisions, develop new behaviours and eventually, move towards the life of your dreams.

A final thought is to never forget that this is just a roadmap. There are certain things that could happen when you use any map to travel towards your destination. Remember to be kind to yourself when you sometimes take the wrong turn, run out of fuel or even screw up big time while trying to overtake the villains on the road. When you slip or things go wrong, stay in the comfort of knowing that you have a clear map and you know where you're headed. And none of this has to be cast in stone. If your destination and your goals change altogether, you can always change your storyline and make it end differently.

153

FOUR WAYS TO DEVELOP NEW BELIEFS

When I conduct training or coaching sessions for clients, one of the things that I almost always have to deal with is helping clients develop new beliefs. A person who believes in his or her potential to change and develop is infinitely more likely to produce desired results than a person who does not. It doesn't matter what you're trying to achieve. Losing weight, finding a new job, attracting your ideal life partner, getting paid more or even trying to find peace of mind or becoming happier. If you'd already believed strongly enough, you would already have achieved what you wanted in that area. You're sure to be more in need of belief, in an area of your life where you are struggling to achieve your goals and live the life you want. Here are four methods that have helped a lot of my clients and they're bound to work for you. These are unlike the usual suspects of writing down your goals or visualising them.

Spend Time with People Who Believe

Going beyond clichés like "birds of a feather flock together" and "you are the average of the five people you spend the most time with," there is some truth in the amount we might absorb from the people we hang out with. So spend time with people who already have the kind of beliefs that you're trying to develop. If you're trying to run a marathon, go join a runners' club and get into the circle of people who've already run a couple of marathons. You're bound to pick up their vibes, their vocabulary, their habits and eventually their beliefs.

Flood Yourself

Imagine you are down with a virus and are going to meet a new doctor. What would make you feel better? Hearing success stories of the number of people the doctor has cured or hearing of the number of people who have got worse after meeting that doctor? In order to build your belief in a particular area, flood yourself with supportive information by reading books, watching videos or even talking to people who tell you things to strengthen your belief rather than weaken or even shatter it. If you joined a martial arts class after watching a documentary on martial arts and getting inspired by the health and wellbeing benefits of martial arts, then do things to keep that flame alive. Read articles about the health benefits of martial arts, watch some more documentaries or even take some seasoned martial artists out for lunch or dinner and understand how the art has helped improve their lives. Remember to club this approach with common sense. So be realistic and do what works in the circumstances of your life.

Do At Least One Thing Every day

Don't underestimate the power of action. Belief and action almost feed on each other. Do at least one thing every day that will add to your belief. If you are trying to learn a new language, learn at least a few words in that language a day or look up what courses are available in your city, or get in touch with a person who can teach you that language or even buy a book or download a language-learning app. Any of these will take you a small step closer to your goal. Each time you do this, a small ounce of belief is built in your system. With each tiny increase in your belief, the more likely you are to take more action and eventually your belief and your action will nurture each other to drive you forward.

Don't Be Obsessed

There is something about being desperate to achieve your goal that causes your goal to evade you. People who are passionate about something have a positive outlook towards what they're trying to achieve. On the other hand, people who are obsessed about something are almost functioning from a place where they feel failure is imminent. I've often seen people desperately trying to get married, desperately trying to have kids, desperately trying to make money and some even desperately trying to get happier, and it never works. Don't let your entire life start revolving around the one thing that you don't have in life because you don't have supporting beliefs in that area. Take steps towards building new beliefs but don't forget to continue living your life and enjoying the things that you already have.

If after following the above four tips, you're still struggling to develop new beliefs, then you might want to sit back and think about whether you actually want those beliefs. The reason you might not believe that you can buy a mansion in an elite neighbourhood could be because, in your heart, you don't actually want to go live in such a neighbourhood. The reason you don't believe that you can get a higher paying job might be because way down inside, you don't want to work any harder or take on more responsibilities. The reason you don't believe that you can recover completely from a health problem is likely to be because the health problem is your perfect alibi for your underachievement in other areas of your life.

MENTAL GAMES OF WELLBEING

A SNAPSHOT

The World Health Organisation's definition of health as contained in its constitution is "Health is a state of complete physical, mental and social wellbeing and not merely the absence of disease or infirmity." This chapter examines the physical dimensions of wellbeing in terms of fitness and exercise, the mental sides of it in terms of how we perceive and deal with our wellbeing and then the integration of the two into our everyday activities for a good life. My observations on human behaviour especially in terms of the games people play are highlighted here. There are a lot of games that we play every day, and I'm not talking about tennis, basketball or billiards. Nor do I want to allude to Dr. Eric Berne's concept of games.

The games I'm talking about here are ones that we play with ourselves, and they could particularly have a negative impact on our wellbeing. They are patterns of behaviour that surface time and again and in different ways in any man's journey to wellbeing. Bruce Lee said, "Absorb what is useful, discard what is useless and add what is specifically your own." That's what I urge you to do in this chapter, get a glimpse of what some games might look like and check if you might be playing them yourself. Finally, if you still want to play games, learn how to play a few of them right so that they add to the quality of your life.

FEELING BETTER BY PUSHING UP YOUR NEUTRAL LINE

Ask yourself how you feel right now on a scale of one to ten. One being horrible and ten being awesome. Now how do you feel today in comparison to some other days, on the same scale? You could extend this inquiry into an assessment of how you feel this week, this month or even this year. We all have days that are a ten or even a fourteen, and sometimes there are days that are a one or zero. Though it's absolutely normal to experience these highs and lows, the larger question is, "Where do you spend most of your time?" I mean towards which end of the feel-good scale?

The Neutral Line Phenomenon is a concept that I've used, to process the responses to some of the above questions and to help my clients live a happier and more fulfilling life. The Neutral Line Phenomenon refers to an imaginary line that lies in between the high and low states of your life. It indicates your habitual behaviour or your customary state. Someone, who at any given point of time feels they are at a ten, probably has a higher neutral line compared to someone who on most days feels they are at a one or two. While one, two, ten or even fourteen are just numbers on an imaginary feel-good scale, the neutral line is real. It is your habitual behaviour or state and in turn is a true assessment of the kind of life you're leading. People who live an awesome life are actually the ones who feel like a million dollars most of the time. While the people who are going through a mundane existence or even living a life of struggles are the ones who are feeling hopeless and miserable most of the time. There's absolutely no point having a high net worth, being on the cover of Time magazine, taking fancy vacations, getting to the top of the corporate ladder or even retiring at thirty if you aren't feeling good.

You've had a pretty lousy year if you spent the whole year working a job that you hated and doing other things that you were forced to and that you hated yourself for, just to take that ten-day international vacation in December. What this does is that it puts your neutral line way close to the zero mark. On the other hand, if you at least did that lousy job for just five days a week but had a blast during the weekends doing the things that you absolutely looked forward to, then that immediately puts your neutral line closer to a four or a five. Now imagine that you were doing a job that you absolutely loved from Monday through Friday and you had other interesting passions that you spent your weekends being involved in and to cap it all, you also took that lovely vacation at the end of the year. That is when your neutral line is probably inching close to the ten mark. I'm sure you get the picture. The point is to push up your neutral line. Rather than aim for those isolated high times of your life that are far and few between, do what you can to feel good more often and to increase the intensity of that feeling.

Someone whose neutral line is at the happy level, on good days feels happier and on great days feels elated. While for someone whose neutral line is at the depressed level, even the great days are just less sad days.

I want to leave you with a quick and easy exercise to push up your neutral line. It's called 'Just Keep Checking.' I believe that most of our actions are essentially driven by positive intentions. Most people aren't trying to do anything because it's going to help them feel bad. Everyone, by and large are trying to feel good or at least do things because they believe it's going to make them feel better. I feel this even about the people who contemplate suicide. The ones who choose to kill themselves do so because they actually think it's a better option. That's exactly why this exercise works.

Here's all you need to do. Every hour, through the day, from the time you wake up in the morning till you hit the bed at night, just keep checking with yourself how you feel on the imaginary one to ten scale; one being lousy and ten being elated. It doesn't matter where you are on the scale and nor do you need to do anything in particular to change your state. Just keep checking. If you want to, you can even set an alarm initially to remind yourself every hour. Once you've checked and given yourself a score, then just go back to what you were doing. What this exercise does is that it builds your self-awareness. You start to become more sensitive to the way you feel and start to have a sense of where your neutral line lies. If you notice that for way too long you aren't at the end of the scale that you'd like to be in, then it forces you to do things that will push up your neutral line.

THE BLIND SPOTS OF WELLBEING

A piece of news I once read in the New York-based Syracuse New Times website read[33],

"On Sept. 28, 2015, a couple from Syracuse witnessed a grey, circular UFO. Ethan and his wife, Shemlynn, were driving on Interstate 81 south and were about nine miles south of the Watertown exit. The couple said that the sky was overcast, with little sunlight still out.

'All of a sudden, Shemlynn pointed out a grey mass in the sky,' he said. 'The UFO was circular shaped, and it came twisting out of the clouds for about five to ten seconds, then receded.'

Shemlynn said that when the UFO came out of the clouds, it seemed unstable or like it was experiencing turbulence."

What's interesting is that no website or newspaper or TV channel reports the thousands of other couples who were having a quiet evening in New York on that same evening, or for that matter anywhere else in the world. Likewise, if there's one flight that crash lands in some city somewhere, it becomes news the world over while the millions of flights that land perfectly go unreported.

This is what I call the Vital Incident Prejudice. It's a phenomenon that applies to various areas of life, especially to wellbeing. Even in the sphere of wellbeing, it's always the hits that get registered while the misses don't. Start noticing this in your own life. Here are some instances of the Vital Incident Prejudice that you might relate to.

I recently met a gentleman in his mid-fifties, who'd been following a particular kind of vegetarian diet for most of his life. He got to know a month ago that he was diabetic. He's now trying to change everything about his life from his job to his leisure activities and quite naturally, his diet. The fact that the diet he followed all these years helped him stay hale and hearty till his mid-fifties somehow seems to have zero significance all of a sudden. The single incident of being diagnosed with diabetes could make a person throw away something that was a way of life all along.

Look closely at the same example of the man in his fifties. The Vital Incident Prejudice is also at play when he plans to make changes in his life without realising that all he has now is diabetes. He's free from a range of diseases that other less fortunate people in this world are victims of. Examine your life and see if you've been doing this. You could be in the habit of focusing all your attention and energy on that one area that isn't working well in your life. This often happens at the cost of all the other areas that are working perfectly for you. This is known in psychology as the negativity bias[34].

The number of instances of this is endless. People scrapping an entire workout because the instructor made a negative comment about it. People latching on to the one small negative idea in a two-hour conversation that had a sea of positive ones. On the brighter side, there are also people who've quit smoking altogether because they read an article about the link between smoking and impotence or dementia.

Do this. Take a look at all the things that are working well in your life and start by consciously feeling grateful for them. If you're reading this book, then chances are that you already have a lot to be grateful for. It's all those things that make up your overall sense of wellbeing. If something's not going your way, spend some time and energy to fix it but move on. Don't change your entire life around to nourish the plane crashes and the UFO sightings of your life.

THE INVISIBLE DUMBBELL

While there simply is no substitute for a gym or real fitness equipment, you can get as good if not a better workout by exercising the exact same muscles in the same fashion. This is done by applying what's called the 'Invisible Dumbbell' concept – imagining yourself using the weight or fitness equipment in the exact same manner and actually flexing the relevant muscles. Visual Motor Behaviour Rehearsal developed by Suinn[35] (1972, 1994) and the interesting ideas of Dr. Denis Waitley on Visual Motor Rehearsal[36] (popularised through the film *The Secret*) go on to show that even when Olympic athletes ran a race only in their minds, the exact same muscles got fired in the same sequence. The mind actually doesn't see the difference between a real event and you imagining it. If you imagine yourself squeezing one half of a big, yellow, juicy lemon into your mouth in great detail, your mouth will actually begin to salivate. That saliva is real, though the lemon is only in your imagination.

Now stand up and imagine holding a pair of dumbbells, one in each hand. Do it. Carry them like they are really heavy (as heavy as you can handle). If you're carrying these invisible, heavy dumbbells right, you'll notice that you're working the exact same muscles that you would have been if you were carrying real dumbbells. Now begin to do bicep curls with the invisible dumbbells in each hand, believing and acting like you are doing them with real dumbbells. Once again, if you are doing this right, you'll notice that your stance, body posture and even facial expressions will begin to match that of a real dumbbell workout. With each rep, you'll begin to see how your muscles feel the strain.

The many advantages of the invisible dumbbell include being able to get a good workout without straining your back, not having to rely on a gym or actual equipment and being able to work out even when travelling, since your invisible dumbbell will breeze through airport security checks. The concept of the invisible dumbbell can be extended to other kinds of fitness equipment if clubbed with common sense. You could also have the invisible barbell, the invisible bull worker, the invisible jump rope, etc. but certainly not the invisible exercise ball or the invisible inclined bench. Importantly, this isn't just about an invisible dumbbell. It could be about anything else in life.

If what makes you feel relaxed is lying back on a recliner on the beach and listening to the sound of the waves, then try and reproduce the same thing at home. Recline in your bed or sofa, close your eyes and imagine you're at a beach. You can make this as real as possible by playing wave sounds on your phone or laptop, switching the cooler on for the breeze and even making yourself a real Margarita or Caribbean Rum Punch if you like. What's invisible here is the beach. If you find all this too much work to help you relax, at least do this. Close your eyes and imagine being at a time when you were completely relaxed. That helps too. You could be in a taxi, going for an important meeting. But imagining yourself sitting on your couch on a lazy Sunday afternoon reading a book will actually make you feel more relaxed.

It's a common predicament among people who try this, to find it slightly awkward and strange in the beginning. But with some mental effort and regular practice, you'll be able to get results that are close to if not as good as ones with the real thing. In fact, holding an actual dumbbell in your hand gives you the luxury of switching off mentally and letting your body do the work. With an invisible dumbbell, you simply need to be more mentally engaged. A thorough and impactful workout is both a physical and a mental game.

The Western school of thought has always been about "First See and Then You'll Believe," while the Eastern school of thought has always been about "First Believe and Then You'll See."

HOW MUCH DISCOMFORT CAN YOU HANDLE?

The clichéd "Comfort Zone" that's so often referred to in self-improvement books and motivational talks, is a space that is defined mostly by our limiting beliefs, past programming and self-created boundaries. When one steps out of this zone, the feeling of discomfort was nature's way of warning early man of a prowling tiger or other potential danger. The rush of adrenaline that followed was to help us attack or run away to save our lives.

In the 21st century, the mantra is **Feel The Discomfort But Do It Anyway**.

This ability to handle discomfort is a recurring theme in anyone's quest for a good life because it shows itself up in several areas. For starters, merely shifting from an unhealthy diet to one that is healthier (and perhaps less tasty) is a challenge for many, primarily because it requires them to put up with a certain level of discomfort. Building any new routine of any sort is another classic example of an initiative that is punctuated with moments of discomfort. This could include waking up early, stepping out of your house on a rainy evening for a jog or even just getting yourself to practice yoga at home after a tiring day.

Unfortunately, there are no shortcuts to dealing with discomfort, obviously because shortcuts are mostly easier and more comfortable. But practising the following two techniques will greatly help in expanding your comfort zone.

The first is what I call 'Embracing Discomfort.' It's during your moments of discomfort that you're actually growing. Many individuals get comfortable with a particular set of exercises or routines and don't move beyond that. Though, real growth happens only when you actually step into your zone of discomfort. It's the extra ten push-ups that you do beyond your comfortable range that actually tones your body more than the initial ones. The entire purpose of any exercise is to get your body to move beyond its sphere of comfort and allow your muscles, your strength and your endurance to grow in the process. So the next time you step out of your comfort zone, be assured that you are making real progress.

The second technique is called 'Revisiting.' Don't stay away from something that has caused you discomfort in the past. It's essential that you use your willpower and resolve to push yourself to visit that same level of discomfort again. The beauty of doing this is that with repeated visits you'll start to realise that what was once "very uncomfortable" becomes only "slightly uncomfortable" and finally moves on to being "totally comfortable." When you see this happening, realise that you're literally expanding your comfort zone.

I've helped people follow this approach to make progress, not just in the area of fitness but in all areas of their lives. The secret to accomplishment is – Get Comfortable with Being Uncomfortable.

WHEN IT COMES TO COMFORT ZONES – SIZE DOES MATTER

The quality of your life is directly proportional to the size of your comfort zone. So what else is this comfort zone all about? The word 'comfort' could mean different things, like a sense of relief, being free from any sort of pain or anxiety or quite simply, being at ease. The space where you experience this relief or freedom or ease is called your comfort zone. In other words, the circumstances, scenarios, places and activities that keep you comfortable make up your comfort zone. Expanding this comfortable space of yours has a huge correlation with various aspects of your life like personal growth, learning, health, wealth, relationships, life satisfaction, etc. Let me outline a few to spell out this point.

Health

After a point in life, being healthy is directly related to how healthy your habits are. If you're only comfortable eating junk food every day and not exercising, you're likely to become obese and unhealthy. To get healthier, you need to eat healthy and develop healthier habits like exercising regularly rather than drinking excessive amounts of alcohol and smoking. Eating green and juicy vegetable instead of junk food, drinking more water instead of alcohol and quitting smoking could be extremely uncomfortable for many. But that is exactly where you need to push yourself beyond your current level of comfort and expand your comfort zone. By consciously doing the things that you might be uncomfortable doing at first but that are good for health and wellbeing, you will gradually expand your comfort zone and in the process step into a healthier life. The key is to make one small and almost unnoticeable change instead of trying to change your whole life around.

Wealth

Your earning potential is directly linked to the size of your comfort zone too. Across organisations, the people who get paid more are the ones who do more complex things and own and execute greater challenges. A lot of people don't grow in organisations because they are not comfortable taking up larger responsibilities and therefore don't get paid higher salaries. There are numerous examples of people who've inherited a huge amount of wealth from their parents or relatives but whose comfort zones were way too small to handle it. Eventually, such people would at best stay where they are and not grow any richer, and if they are unwise, even end up worse than where they started off from. One of the quickest ways to get rich is to expand your comfort zone. Get comfortable with taking greater risks, owning larger responsibilities and working harder than you now think possible for yourself.

Happiness

While there are several things that make a person happy, I'd like to focus on personal growth and fruitful relationship for the moment. One of the biggest causes of unhappiness is having problematic relationships with your family, friends, colleagues or life partner. The most difficult people to get along well with are the ones who think their way is the only right way of being or doing things. Which means such people are not comfortable with any behaviour or interaction from others that doesn't match with their own ideal ones. Developing more harmonious human relationships means being comfortable with different kinds of people, different kinds of interactions and attitudes of others. Being flexible is really just about having a larger comfort zone.

Another big factor that gives people happiness is learning and, in turn, personal growth. Learning anything new involves moving from what you already know and are comfortable with to something that you don't know and need to start getting comfortable with. This is well understood by anyone who's learnt a new musical instrument, a new language or even picked up a new area of work. The very term 'personal growth' refers to growing as a person, beyond your comfort zone.

WELLBEING LESSONS FROM MARSHMALLOWS

Before I start an explanation of the relationship between marshmallows and fitness, I must clarify straight away that eating a lot of marshmallows will not make you any fitter. On the contrary, the gelatin and sugar in marshmallows could take away from your level of fitness if eaten in excess.

So what's the connection between fitness and marshmallows?

In the late 1960s and early 1970s, Professor Walter Mischel[37] did a series of studies at Stanford University to study the phenomenon of delayed gratification. One of them was known as the Stanford Marshmallow Experiment[38,] and it has led to groundbreaking findings and applications of delayed gratification. The experiment was conducted on a group of children between the ages of three-and-a-half and six. Each child was taken into a room by the researcher and given a marshmallow. The child was given two choices. Either to eat the marshmallow right then or to wait for fifteen minutes in the room without eating the marshmallow whiles the researcher stepped out of the room. If the child managed to do the latter, then when the researcher came back, the child was given two marshmallows. Though over

600 children went through the experiment, only one-third of the children were able to delay gratification long enough to get the second marshmallow. Follow-up studies of the Stanford Marshmallow Experiment have also shown that the children who were able to delay gratification went on to become adults with higher levels of academic and professional success, better physical and psychological health as well as greater social competence. The choices are simple, a smaller reward right now or a larger and better reward later. That is precisely the lesson to learn from the marshmallow experiment.

Delayed gratification is the key to greater wellbeing. Fitness particularly is an area that calls for long-term thinking. Many succumb to the lure of an extra hour of sleep, an extra helping of their favourite dessert, an evening in front of the television or the endless excuses of life's responsibilities and social commitments. These instances of momentary excitement and instant satisfaction are a huge trade-off on your long-term health and wellbeing. There is no such thing as short-term wellbeing. Wellbeing must always be approached with a long-term mindset. Waking up early on a cold winter morning to go for a run, hitting the gym at night after a long and tiring day at work, sticking to your exercise routine on a weekend when you'd rather laze around all day or doing those ten extra push-ups that could make your arms and shoulders hurt. All these are equivalent to the child sitting in front of the marshmallow without eating it. The result, as the experiment showed, is getting two marshmallows instead of one. This equates to losing more flab, getting leaner, stronger, fitter, improving your overall wellbeing and being less prone to illness and injury.

As seen in the follow-up studies of the Stanford Marshmallow Experiment, practising delayed gratification will not only ensure long-term health and wellbeing but will also help you develop the right mindset and mental horsepower to successfully deal with the other challenges in life.

GUILT TRIPS AND FITNESS

It's common for people to feel guilty at some point or the other about something related to wellbeing and fitness. On the one hand, you have people feeling guilty because of something they did or are likely to do, like oversleeping, eating an extra cheeseburger with fries, smoking too many cigarettes, etc. On the other, you have the ones who are guilty of something they did not do or are likely to avoid doing, like missing a morning run, not eating enough veggies, skipping medication, etc. Obviously, these are just versions of each other.

For greater wellbeing, people need to choose activities that they really love or at least find ways to enjoy improving their level of wellbeing. Even the clichéd "Fitness is a journey and not a destination" suggests the importance of the process over the final goal in fitness. A guilt trip, on the contrary, could make your entire fitness journey an arduous one.

If you plan to deal with your guilt trips head on, then practice the techniques below.

Quick Reflection

Only you and your conscience know whether or not what you feel is guilt and if your feeling of guilt is justified. The idea is to reflect as soon as you sense the slightest possibility of a guilt-related feeling. Many a times, things start with a feeling of slight discomfort, then it moves on to feeling bad, which moves to feeling heavy inside and if still unattended, moves on to feeling guilty. The idea is to catch yourself before you go all the way there.

Ask Yourself

- ❖ Are you actually feeling bad about not going for a walk or about letting your walking friends down?
- ❖ Are you actually guilty because of what you did or are you just supposed to be guilty? (Many of us function based on habituated patterns that later become our reality).
- ❖ Was not going to the gym the best thing that you could have done that day?

Often, this straightaway redirects you from starting a guilt trip into addressing the issue head on. The idea obviously is not to be at the gym instead of your best friend's wedding or at the cost of your child's admission process. But for that level of moral clarity, it's important that you reflect and reflect quickly.

Different Tips for Different Trips

If you classify guilt trips on a timeline, you might end up with three types of guilt; and obviously, each type needs to be dealt with differently.

❖ **Future Guilt**

Are you one of those people who feels guilty about something that is yet to happen? Like feeling guilty about the aerobics classes that you will miss a week later when you are on vacation or feeling guilty because you know you are likely to overeat at a dinner the next evening. A smart workaround is to plan what I call a neutraliser. Cut down on your calorie intake a little for the next five days to make up for the heavy dinner. Go for a run or swim while you're on vacation to make up for the missed aerobics classes. Just knowing that you have a neutraliser planned, dissipates the guilty feeling.

❖ **Present Guilt**

If you are guilty about something that is happening right now, do something about it. Take action. Move your arse. For example, if you are guilty about reading this book right now, put it down and go do what you think you ought to be doing.

❖ **Past Guilt**

For guilt that haunts you from the past, ask yourself if there is anything that you can do right now to make things better. If yes, then go ahead and do it. If your large paunch or muffin top reminds you of how you let yourself gain weight over the years, then register for a weight-loss programme right now rather than put it on your to-do list. You could perhaps have a light salad for dinner as a neutraliser for the overloaded pizza or stake that you had in the afternoon. But don't just think and waste time, take action.

Guilt Trips and Feedback

Sometimes a health and fitness related guilt trip is trying to tell you something more fundamental about yourself that needs attention. Maybe you are a perfectionist in all areas of your life including fitness, and that needs to change. Maybe you binge ever so often because of a chemical imbalance in your body or a deficiency that needs to be addressed. Maybe you need to deal with failure or underperformance better.

In conclusion, if none of the above work for you, use the feeling of guilt as a negative reinforcement to change the very behaviours that caused you to feel guilty in the first place. Affirm positively or write it down or, at the very least, see yourself getting that behaviour right the next time around.

FIT FOR NOTHING

One of the questions that rarely get asked is, "Why do people need to be fit?" Though this might have been a passing thought in the minds of many, the reason that this question is not asked often is because of the unsaid understanding that fitness is a means to achieve certain other goals like good health, a long life, to have fewer doctor visits, to feel good, etc. Even the idea that some have, of it being too late to start pursuing fitness comes from the mindset that one needs to get fit to in turn achieve some other larger goal like look better, battle a disease, overcome a health problem or win an event and experience a sense of achievement. In reality, fitness is not just a "means goal" that will get you somewhere; it's an "end goal" in itself. This is what I call the 'Fit For Nothing' mindset. You don't have to get fit to feel good; you can feel good while you're getting fit. You don't have to wait till you reach your ideal body weight to feel elated; you can feel elated on your journey to your ideal body weight.

The super fit seem to understand this idea much better than people lower down in the pecking order. Though the extremely fit individuals might have started their fitness journey with a specific goal in mind, most of them continue to pursue fitness well past the achievement of that goal because by then they've already realised that fitness is a way of life and the goal was just another milestone. They pursue fitness for the sheer joy of pursuing it. Anyone who has followed a path of fitness long enough knows that after a certain point, the focus almost always shifts to the experience of the activity. It's quite common for seasoned martial artists or marathoners to talk about practising the art purely for the experience or running for running's sake.

Let's not forget that fitness is an area where the dropouts clearly outnumber the ones who stay. Having the 'Fit For Nothing' mindset greatly increases your chances of following a path of fitness and not quitting. Doing something without expectations greatly reduces the chances of disappointments that arise from not achieving goals and in turn reduces the dropout rate. Having this mindset also helps people see every positive outcome of a fitness regime as a bonus rather than being flooded with dissatisfaction when the planned weight-loss targets or running speeds are not met. One such positive outcome is that any form of exercise causes the release of chemicals like the brain-derived neuropathic factor that reduces symptoms of depression and the neurochemical serotonin that is a great mood enhancer. Exercise also causes endorphins to be secreted in the brain and the nervous system that reduces stress, relieves pain and creates euphoric feelings.

If you approach any form of fitness with the 'Fit For Nothing' mindset, you will enjoy the fitness activity more as you're bound to have fewer negative and more positive feelings associated with the activity.

WELLNESS AND
WELLBEING PHENOMENA

A SNAPSHOT

If you are on a drive to improve your wellbeing, what's the one thing that you must do? A lot of people I've asked this to, talk about something physical like running, working out at a gym, walking, cycling, aerobics, etc., while some others speak about something to do with the mind, like meditation, writing their thoughts down every day, prayer, visualisation, etc. There are also people who've just said, "Well, I don't know. I've never thought about it." This just shows how our biggest approach to wellbeing could vary from what others around us think. Some might not even have an approach. Even wellbeing as a field has a life of its own. There are some inherent qualities that are related to wellbeing, that portray themselves in the physical, mental and emotional dimensions.

This chapter also talks about some dumb approaches to wellbeing that the world today has resorted to and how a few of us, as subjects of it, lap it up completely and hate ourselves for doing so. You will also see the real underlying challenges of living a better life in any form and how certain qualities of wellbeing blend with or bump against certain fundamental human tendencies in terms of behaviour. In that sense, what you read here will be practical insights about what works and what doesn't work if you're trying to live the good life. It eventually touches upon how some people's way of looking at wellbeing could be fundamentally flawed and how they could think of it differently.

WELLBEING IS NOT A NUMBER GAME

This was a few years ago, at the World Economic Forum in Davos. One of the great spiritual leaders and mystics from India was asked by somebody from the business world about what he was doing at an economic forum. The mystic explained how everyone is directly or indirectly in the business of wellbeing and that's also what brought him there. This is true whether we are working on growing our business, buying more property, travelling to more countries, buying fancier cars or experiencing more prestige. The final destination for everyone is to feel good, and to get to and sustain a greater state of wellbeing. To do this, it's critical to understand the actual texture of wellbeing.

Quality is the fabric of which wellbeing is made. A clear understanding of quality in relation to wellbeing is so vital that in its absence, people aiming for wellbeing might just be lost.

These are just a few instances that highlight how wellbeing is rooted in quality.

The Quality of a Workout

People who are new to working out are slightly more likely to make this mistake. They tend to look at various other aspects of the workout than its actual quality. I've heard people say things like, "I've been working out at this gym for the past three years." The question is, "How often do you actually show up to the gym and workout?" A gym is not an old-school organisation where you make progress merely based on tenure. For those who do show up, how long do you actually spend exercising? I've met a lot of people who say they workout for an hour at the gym every day but actually spend more time walking around between exercises and chit-chatting with others. This is when quality is clearly being overlooked. I've seen a few people who take pride in saying they did a hundred push-ups or fifty surya namaskars at a stretch. That's brilliant if you did them right. The point is, how accurately did you do them? Correctness and precision of an exercise or regime far outweigh the number of reps. Eventually, the quality of the workout translates into the quality of the results that it produces for you.

The Quality of Food

Even those of us who don't consider ourselves connoisseurs of gastronomy understand the importance of quality when it comes to food. There is value in a clean glass of water. There is quality even in just the aroma of certain delicacies. Even the breed of people classified as "volume eaters" don't want to eat large quantities of food that tastes pathetic. Secondly, nutritious food is considered better quality food. Obviously, the fast food and junk food industries have completely missed this point. Another clear breach of quality when it comes to food is people not enjoying delicious and nutritious food because of external pressures. The phenomenon of business lunches and breakfast meetings. Mindful eating and savouring what goes into your mouth is the sensible alternative to this.

Quality of Life

Think about it. Anything that any sensible human being does is directly or indirectly with the intention of improving the quality of his or her life. Unfortunately, some fundamental aspects of wellbeing get missed out quite often. The plight of focusing merely on material success while missing out on the fundamentals of life's satisfaction and happiness. Another big factor that takes away from the quality of life is the process of living just for others. People choosing a career path just because their parents want them to, people working a job that they hate just because it pays their bills and people spending loads of time, money and effort just to look good (for others), rather than actually being healthy and feeling good (for themselves).

These are just snippets rather than the whole story. But what's clear is that wellbeing is not a number game. It's about quality rather than quantity. Most people don't want to live to be a hundred if it means that for the second fifty years of their lives they will be in a coma or in some asylum. Wellbeing is about living a high-quality life by experiencing wonderful emotions like happiness, love and peace with the body, mind and intelligence that you're equipped with. It's about using what you have, to live to your fullest potential and enjoying the process of doing it.

FLY-BY-NIGHT WELLNESS

The core of fitness and good health is the feeling and experience of sustained wellbeing. It's not just about repeating a set of exercises every day. It's about enjoying the process of doing it while achieving and keeping the state of health you want. It's not about going to the gym every day but doing the right things while you're there. It's not about getting on a crash diet and losing a lot of weight but ensuring that you don't gain it all back a month later. Quick-fix solutions and shortcuts seem to be the refrain of today's wellbeing industry. You come across ads that make all sorts of before–after promises that signify the urge to get to better health or look good quickly. These are symptoms of what I call the 'Fly-By-Night Wellness' mindset – the ephemeral approach to wellbeing, which stresses more on the speed of achieving the so-called results rather than the permanence of a solution. One big aspect of the 'Fly-By-Night Wellness' mindset is reducing things to its short-term and easy-to-sell versions. Here are two subsets of this mindset that I've noticed.

The 'Passing the Buck' Mindset

People pursuing any kind of health and fitness activity end up not achieving their results because they pass on the responsibility of achieving their goals to someone or something else. There are many who reduce a fit lifestyle to having a gym membership. The larger question is how often you actually show up to the gym and what you end up doing while you're there. Some take it one step further and not just join a gym but also sign up a personal trainer, as if that is a sure-shot way of reaching their fitness goals. As Jack Canfield, the author of the 'Chicken Soup for the Soul' series and several other books, mentions in one of his talks, "You can't hire someone else to do your push-ups for you." Of course, there are the less enthusiastic who pass on the buck to their walking partners, their dieticians and even their home-fitness equipment.

One fundamental dimension of improving your wellbeing is to take complete responsibility for it and to realise that anything else, like a health club, fitness instructor or even the right fitness gear is only part of a support system.

The Simplifying Mindset

Anyone who's done aerobics, yoga or martial arts realises that it takes a while to understand the various nitty-gritties and nuances of getting different exercises, postures or movements right. Typically, a good teacher or instructor will ensure that the student is doing it absolutely right and therefore reaping the complete benefit and experience of the practice. The simplification mindset sets in when slowly and steadily, critical elements of a practice get dropped either due to the lack of supervision by an expert or due to the trivialisation of certain elements by the students themselves. Over time, this simplification could even lead to an exercise or routine being forgotten altogether until you get reminded of it much later. The phenomenon of focusing merely on the number of pounds of the dumbbell used for a particular exercise rather than the correctness of each movement of that exercise. Or the phenomenon of an artistic and impactful set of asanas like the surya namaskar being reduced to the number of surya namaskars that can be done in an hour.

Another critical dimension of getting into a state of good health and fitness is to value every single element of any fitness regime that you are following and ensuring that it's not diluted over time or reduced to something else altogether.

Good health and wellbeing are not fly-by-night operations. It's not about getting a two-month crash course to become a certified instructor of a deep and profound system, it's about getting to the heart of any practice, however long it takes, experiencing it in its completeness, owning it and then being able to share it with others to help them live better lives. By the way, these are just a couple of examples. Use this to start noticing other fly-by-night wellness areas in your life and your environment and deal with them more effectively.

THE FITNESS DRIFTER

Have you ever heard a person say something like this?

"I did two months of kick-boxing, four weeks of spin classes, joined the xyz gym for a month and now I am doing power yoga, which I love because our instructor also makes us do Pilates once a week."

This is most probably a Fitness Drifter talking. A person who drifts like a vagabond, from one fitness system to another, without sticking on to any. A person who pulls the plug on a fitness programme after the honeymoon phase. Let's face it. For many, wellbeing is not a walk in the park. It's an outcome of copious amounts of directed physical and mental effort. By quitting as soon as you encounter difficulty in a path of fitness, you miss the opportunity to create the desired wellness outcome. Whichever system you follow to keep fit, your real fitness programme starts after the warm-up period. Every fitness programme is exciting at the start; it's when the initial thrill fades away that a person's true mettle is revealed.

How to Stop Drifting and Stay Rooted

1. If you've been drifting, the first step is to become aware and acknowledge it. Many fitness drifters

live in the fond illusion that the actual issue is with their aerobics instructor or their gym's ambience or any other external source. To be able to change a behaviour, it's important that you first accept that a certain behaviour of yours needs to be changed.

2. The next time around, pick a fitness system that interests you enough to stay with it for a long enough period. Treat it like a committed relationship, not a one-night stand.

3. Talk to people who've been practising your chosen fitness area for a couple of years and ask them about their challenges and how they overcame them. Just knowing this will keep you better prepared to handle those challenges if you ever encountered them.

4. Realise that in any fitness path that you take up, there might come a point when you hit the wall. So dropping out of one stream and jumping into another is not the solution. Sticking it out with one path is.

5. Join a fitness regime because of your interest in building your fitness by following the chosen system. This will greatly increase your chances of learning that fitness system, growing with it and getting fitter in the process. Don't join a path just to expand your network, build contacts or meet the love of your life.

6. Get into a fitness class with the mindset of creating and maintaining a new lifestyle or way of living. Not to just follow it for a month or even a year.

Having said all this, I must admit that from a wellbeing perspective, fitness drifters are several notches higher than people who are not into any kind of fitness regime at all. The fitness drifters at least manage to keep the fitness flame alive in their lives. There are also people who get bored easily, and actually enjoy the process of learning a new activity. A new fitness regime works different muscles and poses different challenges. Of course, not every runner needs to be a marathoner. Even working out consistently is a way of staying anchored and not drifting, though your flavour of the month might be a different activity.

AS-IF WELLNESS AND THE SWAN EFFECT

Though most people don't realise this, a big part of the wellbeing industry is based on the idea of reproducing certain wellness results that were produced on one person, for several others. This has given rise to fitness equipment, proteins, certain kinds of exercises, meditations, positive coaching interventions and even specific diets. The whole underlying philosophy is that if someone did something and was able to produce certain wellness results, then the same results should be reproducible in another person if that person was made to do the same things. This phenomenon is called As-If Wellness. This is an idea that has probably been around for ages, and it is exactly why people want to follow the fitness plans and workout methods of icons like Arnold Schwarzenegger and Bruce Lee. The As-If Wellness phenomenon essentially says that if you want to get fit, start by acting as if you are fit. In other words, if you want to be fit, do what fit people do. To understand this better, consider some of these differentiators. Most fit people could have eating habits that are different from that of people who are not fit. A fitter person is more likely to be spending some time pursuing fitness compared to a person who is not fit.

Fitter people are more likely to be able to exercise willpower than people who are not fit

By developing the right eating habits, making the right time investment and being able to exercise more willpower in the right direction, you can move from a lower to a higher level of wellness. Now, these are just three examples, but in reality, there are several more.

So, in case you're wondering what the Swan Effect is all about and how it's linked to the As-If Wellness phenomenon, here it is. If you plan to use the As-If Wellness phenomenon well, you need to understand what the Swan Effect is. All of us have seen swans move gracefully on the surface of water as if they're just flowing along some automatic path. What most of us don't see and certainly don't realise is the amount of hard work and rigorous paddling that goes on beneath the surface. This is called the Swan Effect. The phenomenon of the grace and beauty taking centre stage with the actual toil and driving force under the surface being concealed. To use the As-If Wellness phenomenon well, you need to acknowledge and appreciate the Swan Effect in the sphere of wellbeing.

If you've ever been awed by a movie star's chiselled body, don't overlook the difficulty of following a strict diet, despite hectic travelling and acting schedules. If you want to develop the fitness level and agility of Olympic athletes, also think of the number of early mornings and painful practice sessions that it must have taken them to get there. We are often carried away by the result or the destination and miss out on the journey or the drive that it takes to get there. If you want to be a fitter and healthier person through the As-If Wellness phenomenon, the result is a good starting point because that's what you see instantly and that's what inspires you. To complete the loop, you should certainly develop the desired habits, eat the right diet, spend the required amount of time and go through the grind and practice what it takes to get healthy and fit. That's when the As-If Wellness phenomenon is fully expressed.

FITNESS TIME WARPS

To pursue any kind of fitness, time is a fundamental investment that you need to make, apart from effort and money. Interestingly, this time invested to pursue fitness goes through some fascinating distortions. These are what I call Fitness Time Warps. Understanding and working around these time warps will ensure that we are not trapped by them in our quest for a fitter and healthier life.

Now Is as Good a Time as Ever

People often link the start of a fitness process to other events in life. Whether it is joining a gym, starting a martial arts practice or learning Pilates, people tend to link it up to events in other areas of their lives. Don't wait for the completion of a project to start working out. Don't wait to come back from a vacation to start walking in the morning. Don't wait to find a new job and then start learning kick-boxing.

The Obsession with Round Figures

At the beginning of every year, millions of people around the world make New Year resolutions to start some kind of a workout regime. However, by the end of January, the people who are following any kind of workout regime are most likely to be the ones who were working out even during the previous December. At a slightly micro level, people try to mentally match the start of their workout with the first day of the month, the first day of the week and sometimes even make a mental plan of starting a workout at 6 o' clock, 7 o' clock, etc.

Duration Time Warps

I don't want to sound as if only the people evading workouts are subject to time warps and the fitness enthusiasts are free of them. There are clear time warps that are related to the actual workout itself. Any kind of desperation or struggle causes time to move slower. If you've been working out regularly and are still struggling to lose weight, it could feel like you've been working out forever. Likewise, the extra ten pull-ups or the extra sixty seconds of holding a particular stretch could feel like an hour. On the contrary, when you enjoy your workout, time tends to fly. An hour long run or session at the gym you enjoy can feel like just twenty minutes. Another kind of the duration time warp usually happens if you're used to a particular workout routine. You know the routine so well that you tend to go into an autopilot mode or what is more loosely called a trance, typically causing time to fly.

There will always be other events that start and get over in our lives; fitness should be a parallel and uninterrupted journey. The truth is that as far as fitness and wellness are concerned, every day could be treated as New Year's Day and there is nothing stopping us from starting a fitness regime on the 5th of the month, on Wednesdays or even at 6:35 in the evening. Most importantly, when you do start a fitness regime or are in the midst of it, find ways to enjoy the workout and be present both physically and mentally to get the best out of it.

THE GRADUAL SLIP EFFECT – HOW WE ALL SLOWLY LET GO

There was this incident that a friend of mine narrated to me about the first time she went to live with her grandmother for a week. Now her grandmother was an independent old woman who lived alone ever since she was widowed and on the first day of my friend's visit, there were other guests there too. At the dinner table, on the spotlessly clean tablecloth, there was a spread of delicious food, awesome cutlery, the appropriate wine glasses, hand towels, beetroots and carrots cut in the shape of flowers, also actual flowers on side tables that sent out a wonderful fragrance in the room and so on. The next day there were no guests, and it was just my friend and her grandmother for dinner, but all these arrangements remained. The next day and the next day and the next. So on the fifth day, my friend asked her grandmother why she went through the trouble of making all these special arrangements for dinner even on days when they didn't have any guests. Her grandmother replied, "It all starts with one small slip, my dear. At first, you think the fresh flowers aren't necessary. Then you wonder why you have to cut those carrots and beetroots into designs if nobody else is going to see them. Then you use regular wine glasses instead of goblets. Eventually, even the food you cook gets reduced to the 'easy to cook' and run-of-the-mill dishes until you are finally eating takeaway sandwiches or cup noodles on your couch."

The insight from her grandmother's advice is what I call the Gradual Slip Effect. It is a phenomenon that comes into play only when a person already has an established positive behaviour or habit that gradually starts to fade. It is applicable to wellbeing as much as it is to the overall quality of life and the various dimensions of it. You never move from having a flat abdomen to having a pot belly overnight. The slip happens very gradually. So gradually, that even if you put a camera in front of the person, it'll be weeks before you notice any change. If you're a person who's been working out regularly, it's quite unlikely that you stop cold turkey. You know the Gradual Slip Effect is at work when you move from working out every day, to taking Sundays off, to taking the whole weekend off, to taking a mid-week "recovery" break, to working out at least twice a week to eventually justifying to yourself that if you're working out just once a week, you might as well not do it, and then you quit altogether.

The same is true with the start of various other behaviours including the usual suspects like drinking, smoking and eating junk food. It starts with being a teetotaler (your established positive behaviour), then shifts to being a social drinker, then an "only weekend" drinker, and I think you know the rest. People develop new behaviours (both good and bad ones) gradually. It is a really precious minority that is able to change a behaviour in one shot. The idea is to catch yourself with a slip that could be ever so slight and ensure that you bring yourself back on track before things go spiralling downwards. If you are a calm and composed person who's been noticing of late that you are developing a short temper, then catch yourself when you experience even an iota of an irritation and correct that behaviour before you're screaming your lungs out at someone and burning precious relationship bridges.

By the way, there's no hard and fast rule that you need to work out every single day or that you must drink only socially or even that people must always be calm and composed. That's clearly not what I am saying. People must have the freedom to do what they want to in life. Being aware of phenomena like the Gradual Slip Effect and using that awareness to your advantage help when you really want to develop positive behaviours and healthy habits but are unable to do so.

THE PLACEBO EFFECT IN HEALTH AND WELLBEING

The word 'placebo' in Latin literally means "I will please." It refers to any substance or treatment that is used to please the person rather than have any direct benefit. Though the first significant research on the Placebo Effect[39] dates back to the work of John Haygarth in the 18th century, there are several who have studied the Placebo Effect thereafter, including the popular French pharmacist Émile Coué. The Placebo Effect is essentially the phenomenon where a person experiences some sort of benefit from a fake drug or treatment. The phenomenon of headaches vanishing after the patient is given sugar pills instead of real ones or a fever coming down after an injection of saline water that the patient thinks is an actual shot of Paracetamol.

The Placebo Effect is not just confined to the medical field but is hugely prevalent in various spheres of health and wellbeing both in good and bad ways. In fact, when a neutral substance, treatment or practice produces an adverse effect on a person, it is the opposite of the Placebo Effect and is called the Nocebo Effect. Here are a couple of typical examples of the Placebo Effect that I've noticed.

The Start-Stop Effect

Some people who have just started any kind of workout start seeing imaginary results. The phenomenon of a newbie going to the gym for just two days and feeling his clothes fitting him better or seeing his body in better shape when he looks at himself in the mirror. The exact opposite could occur with people who've been working out for a long time. When they skip their workout for just three or four days, they start to feel like they're gaining flab or losing muscle tone. Obviously, months of working out can't possibly get neutralised in a couple of days and two days of working out can't possibly show visible results.

The Comparison Effect

Another classic phenomenon is one that sometimes occurs when you meet people who are at a different fitness level compared to yourself. A moderately fit person might meet a bunch of fat or obese guys and suddenly start feeling fitter than he actually is. The same moderately fit person might land up at an ultra-marathon or some fitness event that has a host of people far fitter than himself and start to feel less fit than he actually is. This is also what happens when you meet people who eat healthier diets or eat far more junk food than you do. Though in reality, your fitness level or the quality of the diet you've been following and its effects don't change overnight. Of course, a wise thing to do is for you to use this as inspiration to keep going right on with your fitness secret.

The New Information Effect

It's always interesting to note how when certain people hear something about health or fitness, their whole perception of things changes. For example, a person who has been drinking milk all her life suddenly hears from a friend or relative about the fat that is contained in milk and the related dangers. She then starts to not just feel unhealthy but also starts to treat milk like poison. The other end of this spectrum is when a person who has been drinking eight glasses of water for most of her life, reads a piece of research about the correlation between good health and water intake and starts to suddenly feel immortal.

I'm hoping by now you have a good sense of how the Placebo Effect manifests itself in various areas of health, fitness, exercise, diet and overall wellbeing. Spend time identifying your own instances of the Placebo Effect in life and use them to your advantage. By that I mean, using the Placebo Effect to kick-start a workout plan, to start eating healthy, to register for a fitness class or to start a walking or running practice. Not to start drinking more alcohol, to stop working out, to restart a smoking habit or to roll off a healthy diet.

THE MANY SHADES OF HEALTH AND WELLBEING

All too often, people tend to anchor their good health and wellbeing to a specific set of causes or parameters. One popular notion is the connection that a lot of people make between wellbeing and losing weight. Being slim is great, but it isn't the single and only metric of a good life. There's this wonderful movement that first appeared in the 1960s called Health At Every Size (HAES)[40]. It advocated that the changing culture toward aesthetics and beauty standards had negative repercussions for fat people. They believed that because the slim and fit body type had become the acceptable standard of attractiveness, fat people were going to great pains to lose weight, and that this was not, in fact, always healthy for the individual. They contend that some people are naturally a larger body type, and that in some cases losing a large amount of weight could, in fact, be extremely unhealthy for some. Many health and wellbeing enthusiasts are convinced about ideas such as:

- ❖ "Work out for an hour every day, and you'll be fit and fine."
- ❖ "Drink two litres of water a day, and you'll be in great health."

* ❖ "If you don't drink alcohol or smoke cigarettes, you'll live long."
* ❖ "Practice yoga for an hour every morning, and you won't have any health problems."
* ❖ "Shift to a vegetarian or vegan diet, and you'll have more energy."

This is what I call the 'Apple A Day' mindset. It's the mindset that causes people to believe that their health and wellbeing can be reduced to one specific magical variable. Being healthy is the result of a combination of factors; some well within our control and some that are completely out of our control. The converse of the 'Apple A Day' mindset and the more useful one is what I call the 'Way Of Life' mindset. The phrase 'Way Of Life' itself suggests consistency, and it refers to the multidimensional nature of health and wellbeing. A state of good health is the outcome of a number of factors like the right eating and drinking habits, the right amount of exercise, a blessed genetic inheritance and several more factors, many of which might not even be in our popular consciousness. If you drink two litres of water a day and sit in your couch all day long watching television, you're going to be as unhealthy as if you practice an hour of yoga in the morning and spend the rest of the day drinking large amounts of alcohol and smoking sixty cigarettes. The 'Way Of Life' mindset also applies to ill health and disease as much as it does to good health and wellbeing. I've often heard people say things like:

"God! She ate so healthy and never missed her morning walk and exercise, and she still had a heart attack at 40."

OR

"I can't believe that after a lifetime of smoking and eating fatty food, this man is still hale and hearty at the ripe old age of 85."

Statements like these just go on to show that there isn't just one dimension to your health and wellbeing. The 40-year-old might have exercised regularly but could have been stuck in a job that she hated and faced extreme levels of stress day in and day out. On the contrary, the 85-year-old smoker might have been from a family where his parents and even grandparents went on to celebrate their 100th birthdays.

At a time of quick fixes and one-stop solutions, the real perks go to those who realise that merely eating an apple a day might not keep the doctor away if everything else that you do is counterproductive to your health and wellbeing. When it comes to wellbeing, it's not one factor overriding the others, it is each factor working in tandem with all the others, many of which are yet to be uncovered by our scientists and researchers. The future might well shock us by revealing some of the most unexpected factors and their correlation with human wellbeing. While it's impossible to spot every single dimension of your health and wellbeing, a wise approach is to identify the ideal combination of factors that work for you and invest your energy, keeping them under check.

BLISS WITHOUT BAGGAGE

A SNAPSHOT

I've talked so far about certain behaviour patterns of people in relation to spirituality. This chapter talks about what spirituality could be and perhaps what it has not been in the lives of many people. What you read here is hardly what I've learnt through my consulting work or my clients. They're the outcome of two decades of meditation, during which I've meditated almost every single day, and that's something that's made me feel good. But that's just one hour of the day. A lot of what you'll read here is about things I've done and have helped other people do to spread that good feeling to all parts of their day and their lives. The idea of living in bliss as much as you want and answering the question that one of the co-creators of Neuro-Linguistic Programming, Richard Bandler often asks, "How much pleasure can you stand?" You'll also get a glimpse of what really works when it comes to happiness and wellbeing and what doesn't. The other undertone of this final chapter is about moving your arse and taking action right now, rather than saving happiness and wellbeing for your retirement. If you want to experience bliss and happiness, now might be a slightly better time than when you're on your deathbed.

DON'T RUN AWAY FROM BOREDOM

Before I started writing this article, I went on Google and ran a search with the terms 'How to Get Bored.' The results were hilarious. Nine out of the ten results on the first search page were about how to kill boredom. "5 Ways to Overcome Boredom," "17 Things to Do When You Are Bored out of Your Mind" and "10 Ways to Conquer Boredom" were among the search results.

If you have kids at home, you probably hear about getting bored way too often. Though a lot of parents resort to the quickest escape route of handing them the iPad, smartphone, laptop or switching on the television for them. Pop culture today seems to be hooked on to ways of getting rid of boredom with a vengeance. With an endless list of suggestions like meet new people, join a class, travel, develop a hobby, volunteer, do this and do that. Why? What's the problem? It's not a sin to be bored. On the contrary, boredom can be a fabulous way to get more out of life. Here's how.

First of all, boredom helps in sparking new ideas. To mention Robert M. Pirsig[41] again, who was considered to be one of the most widely read philosophers still alive, he said that boredom always precedes a period of great creativity. Another one of his famous quotes on Zen and nothingness alludes to the same thing and it reads, "If you stare at a wall from four in the morning till nine at night, and you do that for a week, you are getting pretty close to nothingness."

Secondly, getting bored gives you the great opportunity of getting more time for yourself. Most often, when you hear people say that they don't have time, they're talking about not having time to do the things that they want to do in life. In a generation that patronises multitasking, getting more done in less time and keeping busy as opposed to living and experiencing a richer life and stopping to smell the roses, many don't realise that getting bored is the opposite of whizzing past life and missing out on it. In fact, I think children should get bored. It's a great way to get them to be more creative and experience time and life in its completeness. The same applies to adults. A lot of adults today don't give themselves even the remotest chance of getting bored. Even a long weekend is filled with activities and things to do, and before you know it, you're back at work.

Third and most importantly, boredom is a sure-shot way to help you look inward. A lot of your goals, visions, aspirations, dreams, likes, dislikes and desires are happening inside of you. All you need to do is look. But if you're so distracted with the world around you and the zillion demands that you put on yourself, then you're bound to drift aimlessly in the high seas. Jim Morrison, the American songwriter and the lead singer of the rock band The Doors, has this wonderful old aphorism[42] about people –

Those who race toward death.
Those who wait.
Those who worry.

Don't be among the ones who race toward death or the ones who worry. Just wait. The next time you get bored, don't reach for your phone, start an activity or schedule new plans. Just wait. Let the boredom set in. Sit through it, experience it, learn to be with it and relish it. You'll get a good glimpse of who you are, what makes you tick and what you should actually be doing in life.

MINDFUL EATING

At a recent conference that I attended on psychotherapy and counselling, I had an interesting conversation with a psychologist who was into Mindfulness-Based Cognitive Therapy. One of the highlights of our discussion was the practice and benefits of Mindful Eating.

We all know that Mindfulness[43] refers to paying attention to your thoughts, emotions and physical sensations and bringing your complete awareness to the present moment. Mindfulness[44] has to do with waking up and living in harmony with oneself and with the world. It has to do with examining who we are, with cultivating some appreciation for the fullness of each moment we are alive. Most of all, it has to do with being in touch. Now if you can do this while you are eating, that's called Mindful Eating. The same is true of drinking, walking, talking or, for that matter, anything else you do mindfully.

Though the brain is capable of taking care of the stomach with respect to hunger and fullness, it's not uncommon to find people who continue to eat even after they are full and people who don't grab a bite despite feeling extremely hungry. The part of the brain, called the hypothalamus controls hunger by regulating energy intake and in turn creating the feeling of satiety. Though most people think that we start feeling full soon after we start eating, it actually takes over fifteen minutes for all the satiety signals to reach the brain. Apart from the satiety aspect, there are a number of other dimensions that determine our eating behaviour, like the quantity of serving, the choice of food, whether accompanied by alcohol or other drinks, our emotional state, the occasion for eating, etc.

What Mindful Eating helps you do is enjoy your food completely and make wiser choices with respect to eating. People claim that they have a problem eating less or dieting because they love and enjoy their food way too much. On the contrary, quite a few of them aren't really enjoying their food while eating it. A typical restaurant or home has people glued to the television, using their mobile phones, socialising or engrossed in conversation while the delicious food is going down their throats incompletely savoured.

Apart from ensuring that you thoroughly enjoy your food while you eat it, Mindful Eating has several other fringe benefits.

The satiety centres of the brain respond not only to the quantity of food eaten but also to the time taken to eat the food. Mindful Eating slows you down, and as a result, you take longer to finish a meal. This will result in you not overeating unnecessarily, which could turn out to be a fantastic technique for weight loss.

Feelings of anger, sadness, irritation or even over-excitement lead to people not tasting and enjoying their food completely. To eat mindfully, you have to slow yourself down and root yourself in the present. This helps in not just enjoying your food more but also establishing more neutral and grounded emotional states rather than extreme ones.

People who've been able to practice Mindful Eating for a while have also questioned some of the other underlying motives behind their eating habits and have been able to address them effectively. What are you truly hungry for? Is it the craving for food or something else that pushes you to eat? Do you eat to meet new people and socialise? Do you eat to get away from your desk at work? Do you eat out of sheer boredom and because you have nothing better to do in your life? Some of these fundamental issues in a person's life can be spotted and addressed as a result of Mindful Eating.

If nothing else, it'll at least help you slow down and smell the roses a few times every day amidst the busy lives that some of us lead.

JUST ONE STEP TO GREATER WELLBEING

We're not left with too many options but to act right now. At this moment. This is true if we're seeking wellbeing or pursuing anything else in life. This includes taking any kind of action, making a decision, putting away a decision, planning for the future, being excited about your goals or even doing nothing at all. The point is that the only moment of power we have is the present. Right now.

Here are two typical behaviours that I've seen in a lot of my clients.

Living in the Past

I was recently called by a gentleman in his mid-thirties who wanted me to suggest a hypnotherapist to him. He was jumping from one health problem to another and suffered from low self-esteem as a result. He perpetually "felt sick" is what he called it. Now this gentleman was not too keen on fixing the problem. In my conversation with him, he told me that what he wanted to do was to go back into the past and find out why he is the way he is. As he innocently put it, "I want to find out exactly why I am like this." So I asked him what he plans to do after he finds out, and he had nothing much to say. As if finding out the underlying reason automatically sorts everything out. So here is someone who lives focusing on the past, wants to blame it and finally does nothing about it.

Postponing the Present

This is another classic behaviour that people demonstrate. The ones who almost live their entire lives chasing a dream, an ideal state of wellbeing or happiness of some form. The kind who say, "Once I've bought that villa, I'll be happy," "After I retire, I'll enjoy life," "After I get my children married, I'll relax," etc. I recently met a slightly overweight manager at an IT firm, and we got down to discussing health and fitness as an important area for goal setting. He said he wants to become slim and run a marathon as well. So I asked him when he plans to start pursuing either of his goals. His response was, "As soon as I move out of this company." I realised that he's been telling others and himself that story through his last five jobs. This is someone who literally teleports what he can do right now into the future by not taking action.

The Point of Power Is the Present

Anything you ever want to change has to be leveraged from the present. In fact, the reasons why you don't sit down and clarify your dreams or break them down into workable plans are exactly the same reasons why you don't achieve them. If you are too lazy to sit and write down your dreams and set milestones, then your laziness might well prevent you from realising those dreams. On the contrary, if you are too busy to take the time out to think about what you actually want in life, then you're likely to not find the time to live into your dream life either. You get the point.

At the risk of sounding like a clichéd 21st-century self-help guru, I want to tell you this. If there is one thing and only one thing you need to do to step into a greater state of wellbeing or to live a better life, just go ahead and take that first step. Right now. Register for that fitness programme, sign up for that marathon or do what you really want to do and experience that greater state of happiness.

You are better off taking that first step right now rather than psychoanalysing the past or fantasising about the future.

SLOW IS BETTER THAN FAST

One of Google's philosophies[45] listed in the "about" page of their website is "Fast is better than slow." Google calls this one of the ten things that they know to be true. That might work perfectly for a corporate giant like Google, but not necessarily for human beings.

I have a friend who went on a weight-loss mission last year. His goal was to get MBA admissions into a B-school in the U.S., and after that, his immediate goal was to drop to below eighty kilograms. He was 103 kilograms when he started and had never dieted in his life, ever. So when he started walking about 10 kilometres every day and went on a strict diet, his body responded phenomenally well. He dropped exactly 24 kilograms in two months. It was an incredible success story despite the fact that the suits and other clothes that he had gotten stitched to take abroad were loose and dangly by the time he left. Here's what happened when he got to the U.S. His workload increased, academics and deadlines took priority, and since he was on a student budget, he succumbed to the quickest escape route of eating junk food. Suddenly there was no time to even sleep, let alone walk or exercise. The long and short of it is that he put on about half the weight he had lost in about six months and the rest of it thereafter. If this trend continues, he'll soon be heavier than he ever was.

'Fast is better than slow' is a great philosophy for the speed of website searches, automobile performance or Amazon deliveries. In the case of health and wellbeing, it rarely works. Of late, I've been suggesting to anyone who's on a weight-loss programme to just focus on losing 1 kilogram a month. This will ensure that in two years you lose 24 kilograms, and this is exactly the kind of weight loss that sticks. What a lot of people don't realise is that a crash diet, quick-fix exercises or workouts and the related plunge in bodyweight are like stop-gap arrangements. To become slim and fit requires you to become a different person – a person with different habits, behaviours and a new mindset. Sudden changes that happen often impact just the physical dimension but leave the mental side of the person untouched. On the contrary, when you lose weight progressively, it means that you've been working out regularly; you've stood the test of time as far as your new diet is concerned, and you've made fitness and exercise a way of life rather than a short-term arrangement.

Now that's just one example. There are tonnes of others. In the travel industry, there is the whole phenomenon of quick travel and package trips. In my view, that's one of the worst ways to see a country or a city and also to approach travel in general. It only works for those for whom visiting places is more of a tick mark than an experience. I recently met someone who went on a package trip to ten countries in fifteen days, and when he was showing me the photographs of his trip on his phone, he could barely decipher one place from the other. In many of the big cities, people are accustomed to rush out of bed in the morning, rush through their morning chores and breakfast, rush to work, rush through their workday, rush back home in the evening, rush to the gym if they're lucky, rush through their workout and get back home to rush to bed. This rushing mindset and lifestyle is the opposite of enjoying life. I also see a lot of people wanting to get rich fast and retire fast, as if work life is a horrible dungeon to quickly escape from.

The real solutions lie in slowing down. As you start imbibing this idea of living a slow and relaxed life, do it slowly. Don't rush into the idea of slowing down. Start by doing one activity every day slowly. Maybe have your coffee tomorrow morning slowly. Very slowly. Make sure you really enjoy every sip of it. Once you've done that, don't be in a hurry to add two activities the next day. Stick with a slow morning coffee every day for a month. If you catch yourself naturally doing a few other things slowly during the month, then good for you. But don't push it. After a month, add another activity. Maybe you can take a slow walk around your block after dinner or read a book slowly before going to bed. Do this for a month and then add one more activity. If you do this, you will begin to notice that you're also learning to give yourself time in other areas of life. If you want to go on a diet, don't change your entire diet overnight. Start with one small change. If you eat four slices of bread, two fried eggs and some butter and jam every morning, then just start by reducing the quantity of butter to half of what you normally eat. Then you can reduce two fried eggs to two boiled eggs. Then keep progressively changing things till you reach your ideal diet.

This is what the 'Slow Is Better Than Fast' philosophy is all about. If you were reading this and thinking that one month is too long of a time or one activity a day is too less of a change, then you are exactly the kind of person who might need this approach the most. Life is not meant to be a speed test; it's meant to be a slow and ornate experience of our existence.

THE REAL ART OF DOING NOTHING

In the consulting work that I do, I now see people realising the downsides of the erstwhile buzzword 'multitasking.' Managers and leaders are now starting to feel that trying to do several things at the same time and at breakneck speed doesn't just have poor productivity and quality implications but also takes a toll on a person's health and overall wellbeing. Quality over quantity is a more meaningful mantra and one that spreads beyond product and service portfolios and into the lives and lifestyles of people.

When I've asked several of these overloaded and often overworked multitaskers of what they really look forward to doing during their breaks or times off from work, I hear a range of things from outdoor adventure to meeting friends for a drink. But one recurrent response that frequents the list is "Doing Nothing." While most of us know logically that it's impossible to actually do "Nothing," it's also true that we know what people more or less mean when they say that. "Doing Nothing" is a great way to increase your sense of wellbeing and experience more bliss in life. It's perhaps the opposite of multitasking and here are a couple of ways in which you can actually "Do Nothing."

Cut Yourself off from Technology

Since it might be difficult for some of us to cut ourselves completely away from technology, start with what is doable. Stop watching television, turn off the radio, switch off the mobile phone or lock up your laptop. If all this sounds impossible, just start with one of them and do it for just one day in a month. You can then move it to two days in a month and so on. The idea is not to become a recluse but to give yourself the opportunity of experiencing the wonderful feeling of nothingness every once in a while.

Slow Down

If the above suggestion seems like a bit of a jump, just try consciously slowing down. If you take thirty minutes to drive to work, leave a little earlier and for a change, just drive slowly to work. If you live in a big city, this might irritate the daylights out of a lot of people on the streets, but that's alright. Because this is about you experiencing the feeling of doing nothing, and not about them. Wake up a little earlier so that you can eat a slow breakfast. Drink a slow cup of tea or coffee or even just a glass of water. Read a book slowly while you enjoy it, or even have a slow shower if you like.

Do What You Love

Interestingly, this is what a lot of people mean when they say "Do Nothing." They mean doing exactly what they want to, for as long as they want to, or even doing what they really love doing in life. When clients I coach tell me that they want to do nothing, I ask them, "Like what?" and they say something to the effect of, "Like take a vacation" or "Like read a book" or "Listen to music" or "Have a long and relaxed brunch with friends" or "Take long walks" or "Lie down by the ocean and look at the blue sky," etc. All of these are specific things to do and yet what they have in common is that they are things that these people really really want to do. So, if you want to do nothing, start with doing what you really love.

Stroll

Get out of your house and take a walk, but aimlessly. We're so used to doing activities with an agenda that we mostly walk only to get somewhere. Even people who go on a morning or evening walk have a mental target of finishing the walk and getting back home. This time, just try walking without any specific destination in mind. Resist the urge to go somewhere as that takes away from the "Nothingness" of the activity. Just stroll around without any specific plan or place in mind. The idea, obviously, is not to get lost but to go with where your instinct takes you and to let your legs guide your direction. Doing this for just thirty minutes is a great way to get a sense of doing nothing.

If the above things don't really work for you, or you think that they're way too bizarre or beyond your control, at least stop multitasking. Try doing just one thing at a time. While driving, just drive. Resist the urge to talk on the phone or listen to the radio. While you eat a meal, just eat your meal, avoid conversations or discussions and while you're reading a book or a magazine, shut off all other distractions.

TWO SURE WAYS TO FEEL HAPPIER

One of the important emotions that people sometimes spend a lifetime pursuing is happiness. There really is a need to focus on "Ways To Be Happy Right Now," as opposed to at any other time or in any other place.

In corporate settings, in families, in academia and, for that matter, in any other walk of life, a lot of people pursue what they pursue, in the end, to feel happy. This approach, I think, is fundamentally flawed and the idea of getting somewhere or earning something or becoming someone and then thinking you will feel happy might deceive you endlessly. The only real way to be happy is to be happy right here, right now. If you aren't happy at any given point in time and that continues, then it's quite like an endless cycle. Moments become hours, hours become days, days slip into months and years and eventually, you're lying on your deathbed thinking how you should have been a little happier when you could.

Our ability to imagine the future could be pretty horrible, especially in terms of what emotions we might experience after we attain a certain state. So I think almost the essential question for someone to answer and get right is how they could be happy right now. Here are just two ways out of many that I know work for sure.

Gratitude

This refers to the things that you are most thankful for and grateful for in life. One of the best ways for you to be happy is to be reminded of all the things that are in your life that you are grateful for. The constant chase of happiness often stems from not being at peace and not being satisfied with where you are in life. It would really help to maintain a folder or notebook called the gratitude journal. By documenting the different things in your life that you are grateful for in this journal, first you make a conscious effort to notice the good things in life. Then, when you take stock of how much you have to be grateful for, you actually start to feel fortunate and happy about it. This process also turns on the reticular activating system[46]. The part of your brain that brings to the forefront the things that matter to you or help you perceive what is important to you. Over time, you will end up with a log book of things in your life that you could feel grateful for. Each time you read this book, it will make you experience the sense of happiness all over again.

Meditation

This is a way of observing yourself in a calm and relaxed manner and not responding to thoughts and ideas that come into your mind. A great way to do this is to sit in any comfortable position, keep your eyes shut and stay focused on your breath. Maintain just a gentle focus on the breath, without making the breath deeper or shallower.

Just the normal breath. If the mind wanders and random thoughts begin to float in, gently focus on your breath again. Don't pass judgements on your thoughts, let them come and go as they will. Be mindful[47]. In the beginning, it might be difficult for someone to observe their breath this way, without responding to their thoughts and ideas. This normally happens for fear of not remembering that thought later. A good way out of this is to keep a notepad and pen handy next to you during the meditation because a lot of what floats through your mind are haphazard ideas, things to do, random memories of the past, random imaginations of future events, etc. Whenever a thought enters the mind that is difficult to ignore, gently open or even half open your eyes, make a note of the thought in the notepad and continue with the practice. This can be reviewed once you are done with the practice, for whatever it's worth. Apart from feeling relaxed or sometimes even feeling happy for no reason at all, meditation helps people see and experience the good things in life more profoundly.

These are just two things that I've used in my own life and helped a lot of my clients and friends use in theirs. This article is only a starting point for future development in terms of accessing the state of happiness more often and experiencing more intense levels of it. Apart from trying out what works for you from the above options, start experimenting with your own approaches to experiencing happiness, document them and practice them regularly thereafter.

LEARN HOW TO SPREAD YOUR LIGHT

For several years now, I've been practising something called "Spreading Light," under the guidance of an organisation called the Manasa Light Age Foundation[48]. It's about imagining a speck of light at what you consider to be the centre of your being, then spreading it to your entire body and then your surroundings and then the entire universe. This is white light that you imagine, by the way. This symbolises to me a phenomenon that occurs all around us and refers to how small changes that happen at a micro level have far greater implications and reach at a macro level than we could possibly imagine. The positive changes that people make in their own behaviour will not just impact them but the people around them, their friends, relatives or colleagues, their environments and so on. This is obviously true even of their negative behaviours.

There are several factors at play when it comes to how we influence one another. One great explanation is through the role of mirror neurons[49]. These are neurons[50] in our brain that cause us to experience what people around us are going through even though we are not directly at the receiving end of the stimuli or situations that cause those experiences.

For example, when we see a person in real life or even on screen crying, we might get teary-eyed or cry. Another big explanation is how we learn and develop new behaviours through the process of modelling others around us. Right from when we are little children, we tend to imitate others and through this imitation, we learn new skills, languages as well as typical reactions to different situations. This is also a way of spreading your light. So what eventually happens is that when you demonstrate a certain behaviour, others around you pick up traces of it and that gets passed on to the people around them, and it's like the domino effect.

Since most of the work that I do is with corporates, an example of 'Spreading Light' that comes to mind is related to the corporate world. There are several companies where the founder or the head of the company is at the centre of the universe that spreads all around him. Richard Branson's adventurous spirit and customer orientation percolates to the entire Virgin staff and even to the policies of the company. The no-leave policy that they launched a couple of years ago gives the employees the freedom to work from where they want and to be on leave as and when they feel like, as long as their work gets done. Likewise, Google that was started by two Ph.D. students from an Ivy League has the practice of taking people who are also from premier educational institutions while Apple that was started by a college dropout boasts of enough examples of artists and poets who built their wonderful products.

My thoughts on 'Spreading Your Light' are mostly related to how powerful it can be as a way to bring about change.

Since you spread both your positive and negative behaviours and mindsets with the same intensity, there is a lot that you can do to ensure that the people and environments around you are positively impacted. If you don't want to do anything else to make your life and the lives of people around you better, at least don't spread negativity. Even doing nothing at all would be a far better contributor.

DON'T POSTPONE LIVING YOUR LIFE

While I was researching a recent wellbeing project, one of the things that caught my eye was how important it is for people to have meaning in their lives. Though, as an idea, this is rudimentary, the number of different areas where the power of meaning is at play is incredible. While this can be comprehended by the amount of importance "meaning" is increasingly being given in the field of psychology, it's also something that most of us understand intuitively.

Here are a couple of things that you can do right now to bring more meaning into your life. The first one is called "Coherence or Congruence." Nothing could be worse than a person being someone he or she is not and living a life that they actually don't stand for. Yet, it amazes me how many people actually do. Quite often, through the corporate consulting work that I do, I find people working for the wrong companies, playing the wrong roles and many who are even stuck in the wrong situations or relationships for years. They just continue doing it because they are used to it, and by now it seems too late to try something different or start something else from scratch. While the work of geniuses like Viktor Frankl talk about how to deal with this, I think there is real value in actually solving the problem by perhaps getting into the job of your dreams or pursuing the kind of life that you actually feel you deserve. While Frankl talks about finding meaning even in a concentration camp, it is important to realise that today we are not in concentration camps and we could actually walk out of our hells if we so desired and planned it well enough.

I'd like to call the second "Near-Death Experience." It's not uncommon for people who've had a near-death experience to come back to life with new zest and meaning. People sometimes see the value and meaning in life only when they've been that close to dying. It reminds me of Steve Jobs's famous Stanford speech[51], where he says, "No one wants to die. Even people who want to go to heaven don't want to die to get there." I recently went to a critical cancer care centre in my city and was surprised to see how many people actually got the counsellors there to call their estranged family members, friends or business partners, so that they could apologise and build a new relationship at least for the brief period that they had left. I hope not all of us will have to wait for a near-death experience or to be diagnosed with a terminal illness to live a more meaningful life.

Start today, by doing the things that matter the most to you. Spend time with the ones you love, take your best friend or relative out for dinner, go for that family vacation that you kept putting away or call up someone you parted ways with for some silly reason and apologise. Because when you are on your deathbed, you'll never regret doing them.

CONCLUSION

As the old saying goes, "You're either at the table or on the menu." If you've reached this far, then you've gone through a menu card of behaviour patterns, insights or methods to change behaviour and improve wellbeing. These are behaviour patterns that I've observed in people I've met through my work, as an organisational development consultant. Especially when I've done executive coaching, life coaching, leadership development and behavioural training. Like in every restaurant, the item on the menu is not the actual dish. You have to order it, the chef has to prepare it, it has to be brought to your table, and you've got to then eat it. At the heart of a restaurant experience is eating and drinking what you love and relish.

After the introduction to this book, I suggested that readers skitter through the book and dip into the portions that catch their eyes and interest them the most. The different phenomena described and the behaviour patterns are all about you. It's what we do as human beings in our daily lives, in our search for wellbeing or our pursuit for excellence. You might have come across several behaviours that you relate to directly and some that you've noticed in others. Now it's time to move from being on the menu to sitting at the table. Do one of the two things that many would do at a restaurant – order what you like and are familiar with or order something that looks interesting, in order to try it out. If you've used something from this book that made sense to you and gave you the results you wanted, then keep at it. If something caught your interest, then try it out and see where it takes you. You never know which dish becomes your next favourite.

Also, having read through so many behaviour patterns, it's high time you start identifying behaviour patterns from your own life and deciphering your own personal take on wellbeing and a good life. Give your life's patterns some names. There's something about naming and defining ideas that make them far easier to refer to, talk about or even think about. Then explore how your understanding of the concept could help you get to what you consider a good life. I recently asked a client to do this himself. This is a guy who loves waking up at 6 in the morning and starting his day with thirty minutes of meditation, doing a few stretches and then going for a forty-five-minute walk. Clearly, quite a health-conscious guy. Being health conscious, he also cares about getting the right amount of sleep. He felt the ideal duration for him was seven hours, and he mostly went to bed between 12 a.m. and 1 a.m. The pattern he noticed in his behaviour was that if he woke up at 6 in the morning, he felt bad that he couldn't sleep enough and his body didn't get enough rest. If he woke up late, he felt bad that he couldn't do his meditation and walk or at least had to skip one of them. The point was that irrespective of when he woke up, he felt bad. He called this behaviour pattern 'Every Morning Blues.' This obviously wasn't his idea of a good life – waking up on most mornings feeling lousy. The moment he spotted this pattern and gave it a name, he became much more sensitive to it when it was happening and didn't take his morning blues for granted. When that happened for too many days in a row, he felt he had to do something about it. Though he's still working on it, he doesn't surf the internet anymore after dinner but reads a book instead. This gets him to fall asleep a lot quicker, and he enjoys many more happy mornings.

If you're one of those people who already lives that life you want to and loves it, then you're probably walking on air and that's awesome. Give that phenomenon a name if you like and hold on to it for as long as you can.

REFERENCES

Introduction

1. Fowers, B. (2011, March 15). Comments on Pascal Bruckner's article "Condemned to joy." Posted to the Positive Psychology listserve: Friends-of-PP@apa.org.
2. William C. Compton & Edward Hoffmann (2013). Positive Psychology, The science of happiness and flourishing, Second Edition. Chapter 12, Page 294.

The Myth About Good-Looking People

3. https://www.cbsnews.com/news/study-finds-attractive-people-earn-more/
4. http://www.telegraph.co.uk/news/science/science-news/10688645/Good-looks-help-you-get-ahead-in-business-if-youre-a-man-Harvard-study-finds.html
5. https://www.inc.com/jeff-haden/oh-great-research-now-shows-good-looking-people-work-better-longer.html
6. http://citeseerx.ist.psu.edu/viewdoc/download?doi=10.1.1.603.5354&rep=rep1&type=pdf

The Link Between Money and Spirituality

7. https://en.wikipedia.org/wiki/Maslow%27s_hierarchy_of_needs

8. http://www.harveker.com/

The "Mine Is Bigger Than Yours" Phenomenon in Spirituality

9. https://thepsychologist.bps.org.uk/volume-22/edition-11/peacocks-tail-altruism

Are Fate and Wellbeing Related?

10. https://en.wikipedia.org/wiki/Nick_Vujicic

Zen and the Art of Decluttering

11. https://en.wikipedia.org/wiki/Pareto_principle

Then What Makes Life Worthwhile – A Snapshot

12. http://www.pink-floyd-lyrics.com/html/free-four-obscured-lyrics.html

Why a Lot of Self-Help Books Hardly Help

13. http://bksiyengar.com/modules/Referen/Books/book.htm

14. https://en.wikipedia.org/wiki/B._K._S._Iyengar

Life Is a Pursuit of Excellence

15. https://en.wikipedia.org/wiki/Robert_M._Pirsig

16. https://en.wikipedia.org/wiki/Zen_and_the_Art_of_Motorcycle_Maintenance

17. https://en.wikipedia.org/wiki/Lila:_An_Inquiry_
    into_Morals

18. https://www.goodreads.com/author/quotes/401.
    Robert_M_Pirsig

Who Is the One Person Who Matters the Most to You?

19. https://www.goodreads.com/work/
    quotes/14746717-politics

Are You Suffering from 21ˢᵗ Century Compassion Fatigue?

20. https://en.wikipedia.org/wiki/Compassion_
    fatigue

Reproducing Excellence

21. https://en.wikipedia.org/wiki/Neuro-linguistic_
    programming

How You Do Anything Is How You Do Everything

22. https://en.wikipedia.org/wiki/William_H._
    McRaven

23. https://www.youtube.com/
    watch?v=pxBQLFLei70

What Moves You to Do Anything?

24. Deci, E.L., & Ryan, R.M. (1985). Intrinsic
    motivation and self-determination in human
    behaviour. New York: Plenum.

25. https://en.wikipedia.org/wiki/Self-determination_
    theory

Wellbeing Doesn't Have to Be a Game of Control

26. http://www.chicagotribune.com/news/columnists/chi-schmich-sunscreen-column-column.html

What You See Is Exactly What You Get

27. https://en.wikipedia.org/wiki/Reticular_formation#Ascending_reticular_activating_system

A Place Where No one and Nothing Can Affect You

28. http://metamorphosiseyou.blogspot.in/2014/07/transforming-your-emotions-zen-approach.html

What Are You Constantly Telling Yourself – A Snapshot

29. https://daringtolivefully.com/tame-your-monkey-mind

What's Your Wellbeing Story?

30. Charles Duhigg, (2013). The power of habit: why we do what we do and how to change. Chapter 3, Page 70.

You Become What You Talk About

31. Richard H. Cox, Sport Psychology, concepts and applications, Seventh Edition. Chapter 9, Pages 224, 225.

Create an Awesome Story for Your Life

32. http://livewritebreathe.com/storytelling-master-walt-disney/

The Blind Spots of Wellbeing

33. https://www.syracusenewtimes.com/ufo-sighting-sept-28-2015/
34. https://en.wikipedia.org/wiki/Negativity_bias

The Invisible Dumbbell

35. Richard H. Cox, Sport Psychology, concepts and applications, Seventh Edition. Chapter 11, Page 282.
36. https://thisconsciouslife.com/2011/06/13/the-power-of-visualization/

Wellness Lessons from Marshmallows

37. https://en.wikipedia.org/wiki/Walter_Mischel
38. https://en.wikipedia.org/wiki/Stanford_marshmallow_experiment

The Placebo Effect in Health and Wellbeing

39. https://en.wikipedia.org/wiki/Placebo

The Many Shades of Health and Wellbeing

40. https://en.wikipedia.org/wiki/Health_at_Every_Size

Don't Run Away from Boredom

41. https://www.goodreads.com/author/quotes/401.
Robert_M_Pirsig

42. http://doors.eu.org/poezje/tapes.html

Mindful Eating

43. https://greatergood.berkeley.edu/topic/
mindfulness/definition

44. Jon Kabat-Zinn, Wherever you go there you are,
Mindfulness meditation for everyday life, Page – 3.

Slow Is Better Than Fast

45. https://www.google.com/about/philosophy.html

Two Sure Ways to Feel Happier

46. https://en.wikipedia.org/wiki/Reticular_
formation#Ascending_reticular_activating_system

47. Jeremy Dean, Making Habits, Breaking Habits
(2013), Da capo press, Chapter 10, Page 154.

Learn How to Spread Your Light

48. http://www.lightagemasters.com/
revolutionbylight.php

49. http://www.apa.org/monitor/oct05/mirror.aspx

50. https://en.wikipedia.org/wiki/Mirror_neuron

Don't Postpone Living Your Life

51. https://www.theguardian.com/technology/2011/
oct/09/steve-jobs-stanford-commencement-
address